WOMBMAN

The Good of a Man, Family, and Society

Ogechi Charity Obayi

*This book is dedicated to my ever-loving and compassionate
Father, for His unending inspiration and guidance upon my life,
and that of my loved ones. And to every young woman who
wants to discover and maximize her life purpose here on earth.*

CONTENTS

FOREWORD

I have gone through this book 'WOMBMAN_ The Good of a Man, Family, and Society' by Pharmacist Ogechi Charity Obayi, it has a total of 13 chapters. The style of writing is so simple and comprehensive, embedded with nuggets to buttress what is been discussed. I believe these nuggets are not just philosophical statements, they are inspirations drawn from Almighty God, given to pharmacist Ogechi. The book is enriching indeed. I have gone through the book and I discovered that emphasis placed on the book if properly harnessed, the Wombman who is the woman will be very good for the man, the family, and for the society at large.

Who should read the book: The first category of person I have noted that should grab the book as a matter of urgency to read because of what it has to offer, we have: No.1. Women of all ages, especially young ladies. It is highly recommended to the woman fork because is going to serve as prophylaxis and as a curative measure. Prophylactic in the sense that there are certain notions women have about themselves which are not correct. So, if a young person, a young lady, a young woman will be able to read this book from page one to the last, it will enable the person never to miss the direction for her life. It is also curative because probably someone might have developed a wrong mindset about women, or herself, as the person read through this book, several things will be corrected so that the person will be able to get live in the right perspective and move on more effectively. No. 2. This book should be read by men also, especially young men because when they read it, they will be able to understand what they need to know about women. You know some men have a very terrible notion or perception about women. So, when they read it, they will be able to understand the true nature of a woman in the plan of God. This book will help change some perceptions some men have about women. Finally, if a man reads this book, he will be able to have the proper knowledge to encourage women; including mothers, sisters, wives, female friends to live to full capacity and fulfill destiny.

In summary, I recommend this book both to women of all ages, and men of all ages. Let me state at this point that the author is not trying to encourage women to rub shoulders with men. She is not in any form trying to promote feminism rather, what she has under God done in this book is to encourage women to see themselves the way God has made them, to see themselves in the right perspective, and be able to move on in line with God's purpose for their life. I needed to say that because if you see the book; some sections with more emphasis on trying to encourage women to see themselves in the true light of how God is seeing them you may start thinking otherwise.

Having said that, the book has been subdivided into 13 chapters, but what the book is generally encouraging women, even men themselves by proxy is to understand the importance of the secret place. The author emphasized so much the importance of the secret place in the life of a woman, and she maintained that the secret place is irreplaceable. A woman who wants to go far in life and become relevant to her generation must maintain a place where she draws strength.

This secret place is a place where you are formed, a place where you receive strength, a place you receive inspiration, a place where you are made, and somehow, it is a secret place; a hidden place, it is more of a personal effort to develop that woman in you. We could see it in two different forms: First, talking from a spiritual point of view, because the book is also backed up by scriptures, the secret place has to do with a place of meeting with God. A woman who has developed the habit of meeting with God her maker daily will be able to develop the substantial capacity to grow and affect her generation positively. Another secret place I'm looking at; the Author is referring to should be a place of personal development capacity building, things you can do beyond what general people are doing to build capacity, develop yourself, and become relevant.

The author continued to emphasize that women should be able to understand and maximize all the intrinsic abilities embedded in them by their builders. I have checked the word intrinsic and it is synonymous with inbuilt. God has deposited something in every woman, God has not left any woman He created without value, without resources, without something. So, the author is beckoning on the women; young and old to read this book to understand some of these abilities that God has put in them and then be able to maximize them. One thing is to understand, another thing is to maximize. If there is no understanding, there will be no maximization.

There are so many intrinsic abilities, remember the wombman is a man with a womb. In other words, women are wired differently from men, they have the attributes of men, and in addition to the conventional attributes of men, they also have some attributes that men do not have; they are men with the womb and so that womb portion is an added value or advantage to women to even explore more and do more than men if they can understand and maximize these abilities.

The author, Pharmacist Ogechi encouraged the readers; women and men alike through the book that they need to understand the need to always go an extra mile in whatever they are doing. For us to affect our generation, the author is insisting that we must not just stop at ordinary things, we must move on to do extraordinary things. She maintained that the difference between ordinary and extraordinary is just the 'extra' there. That we must add and keep adding to what is generally accepted, that we must do extra things to be able to get to a height where we will be able to affect our generation. This book 'The Wombman' talks more about going the extra mile, encouraging men and women to go the extra mile to move very far in life.

Dr. Sunday N. Okafor
(A Lecturer and award-winning Researcher, has published over 40 journal articles in reputable national and international journals, he has reviewed so many articles for many international journals).

INTRODUCTION

We are living in a world where virtually every man and even most women think that being a woman is already a disadvantage. We are living in a world where most women stagger not necessarily because there is no light, but because women have ignorantly refused to discover the woman they are made to be. We are in a world where people assume that it belongs to the men, that the emergence of the woman was an afterthought, that God was comfortable with everything he has created, and later remembered that, there is a need to create a woman.

We are living in a world where the same woman that gives birth to both male & female children is regarded as a lower grade citizen or even someone that is not a first-class citizen. This low view of the woman is more prominent in African countries and is easily evident from the time of delivery. A woman will give birth to a male child and you will hear "she gave birth to a bouncing baby boy" with all vigor and agility in the voice of the announcer. But when she gives birth to a girl, the tune and pitch will be lowered, and the next thing you will hear is "she gave birth to a girl." It left me wondering if the baby boy bounced out of the womb or whether there's a different delivery method for the boy and another for the girl, but I discovered there was none. Then why the discrepancy? Even though no single man on earth came into existence without being brought forth by a woman, yet, this same woman that gives birth to the man is still been regarded as a less important citizen. Without women, the world would have gone into extinction.

Embedded in every woman are some intrinsic abilities that can never be found in men. This is because the presence of the womb in a woman has conferred some qualities that can never be found in any man. Isn't it wonderful to know that as a woman, you are not just a man but a man with a womb? It's like saying that as a woman, you are a man plus womb. It can be mathematically represented as Woman = Man + Womb. So, as a woman, you have the attributes of a man, and also the attributes that the womb confers. These attributes of the womb include the ability to make good, ability to influence, ability to nurture, ability to be a seed carrier, ability to give life to a seed, ability to be perceptive than any other creature, ability to be compassionate and self-denial ability (any woman that truly understands what it means to be a woman, can effortlessly give up many things for the sake of others).

This issue of seeing a woman as a citizen that is of a lower grade, an afterthought of creation, an object of sex and abuse, someone that doesn't have any specific assignment, but is just a helper, was not this way from the beginning. I want to ask you a very sincere question, can you give what you don't have? The office of the woman as a help suitable is beyond just saying that she is a helper! They have the omnipotence of God embedded in them. This is because God does not want to adulterate their helping ability. You can imagine how frustrating it can be to ask for help and you didn't receive it, you can imagine how disappointing it can be when you need help and you confidently asked for such help and the helper couldn't help! This is what God wanted to avoid by putting His omnipotence inside of a woman.

It is good that we make a distinction in this intrinsic ability of the woman to be a help suitable. The fact that she is a help suitable does not mean that she is a help suitable to all men, it doesn't also mean that she cannot be encouraged to help. The helping office of the woman when properly fueled produces a tremendous result that leaves the world in awe. Any wise man that wants to get quality help, must be ready to support the help suitable to give such quality help. This is because she can only dispense the helping abilities you have allowed to be dispensed.

You cannot blindfold someone and expect the person to run effortlessly, neither can you cut the wings of a bird and expect it to fly. Likewise, you cannot subdue the helping ability of a woman and expect quality help. As a woman, when you choose to help someone whom you are not a help suitable to, you will struggle to help and this is never the original plan of God concerning the office of the helper.

God was so deliberate in the making and building up of a woman that He reserved her as the updated and last edition of His creative work. This building-up process of the woman was carried out in a secret place and can only be understood in the secret place. But the problem today is that most women can't sustain the ability to remain in the secret place until they discover this secret in their building up and this has led many women into believing both what is true and what is not true about themselves. This lack of knowledge about the true identity of the woman by most women has led to all manner of competition, insecurities, lack of direction, focus, and other vices. Some women today, in the quest to erroneous feel accepted and to marry because others have married have given in to all manner of vices, some have turned themselves into universal test strip for fertility before marriage. Many women are suffering from all manner of deception all in the name of feeling belonging.

Most ladies today waste their seasons simply because they lack understanding of the times. When you don't understand the season for a particular purpose, you can't fulfill such a purpose, and you end up wasting heavenly resources and you will give an account of it. This is a call for women to understand the times and seasons of their lives. This is time to maximize your God-given abilities as a woman.

In this book, you will understand the importance of the secret place in the life of a woman and why the secret place is irreplaceable for every woman that wants to remain relevant in her generation and also to understand and maximize all the intrinsic abilities embedded in her by her builder. You will understand the need to always go an extra mile in whatever you are doing and not just to remain where others are because what made extraordinary what it is, is not the absence of the word Ordinary, but the addition of the word 'extra.' You will understand the place of time in your season and the reason why you have to prepare at the right time because no matter how good you have prepared in the wrong time, it is as bad as someone who didn't prepare at all. Most women miss out on the season of their lives, simply because they don't understand the times and therefore, never fulfill the purpose of their seasons.

You will understand what it means to be a woman because God made you a woman and not just another man, but a man with a womb. The presence of this womb has given some abilities to the woman, and when these abilities are understood and maximized, it births forth a complete woman that can stand the test of time and live out the original plan of God for women to the fullness.

WHAT HAPPENED TO THE RIB IN THE SECRET PLACE?

And the Lord God caused a deep sleep to fall upon Adam; and while he slept, He took one of his ribs or a part of his side and closed up the [place with] flesh. (Genesis 2:21 Amp)

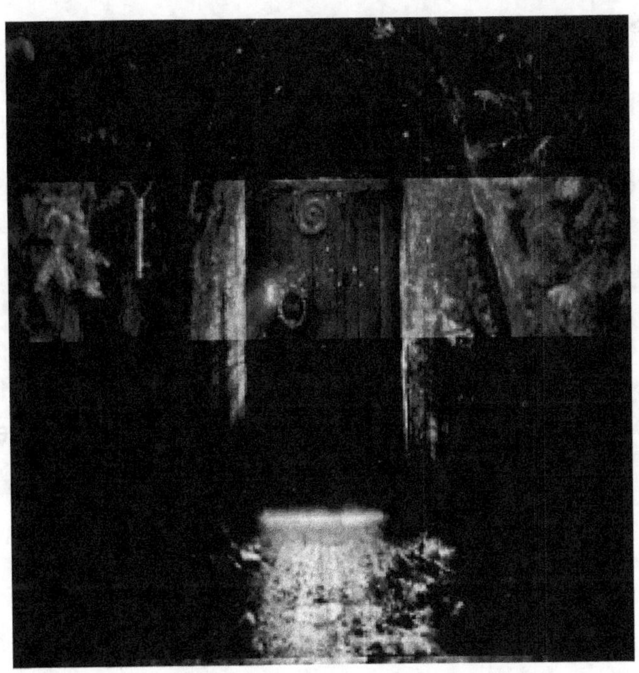

The word "SECRET" means many things, among which includes: Knowledge that is hidden and intended to be kept hidden. Note: It is knowledge but yet at the same time hidden, it is intended to be kept hidden but, the fact that it is knowledge means that it can be accessible; if only you can sustain the ability to subscribe for the knowledge.

"PLACE" could mean many things among which are:

i. A location or position.

ii. A frame of mind.

iii. Somewhere for a person to sit

The word "RIB" *can be any of a series of long curved bones occurring in 12 pairs in humans and other animals...*

"THE SECRET PLACE" to me is a Location or a frame of mind where knowledge that is intended to be kept hidden is unveiled.

The secret place is irreplaceable in the life of a woman because women are formed in the secret place.

The secret place is where we be must be in God, it is a place of unveiling, it is a place of intimacy, it is a place to meet with the Lord in prayer (Communion), it is a place where deep calls unto deep.

Psalm 91:1 made it clear to us that a secret place is a dwelling place. It is a place where weakness is replaced with strength, where solutions are found. You enter the secret place helpless and come out with age-long secrets, ideas, inspirations, and wisdom that when utilized, can change your entire generation.

THE SECRET PLACE FOR A WOMAN IS A PLACE OF:

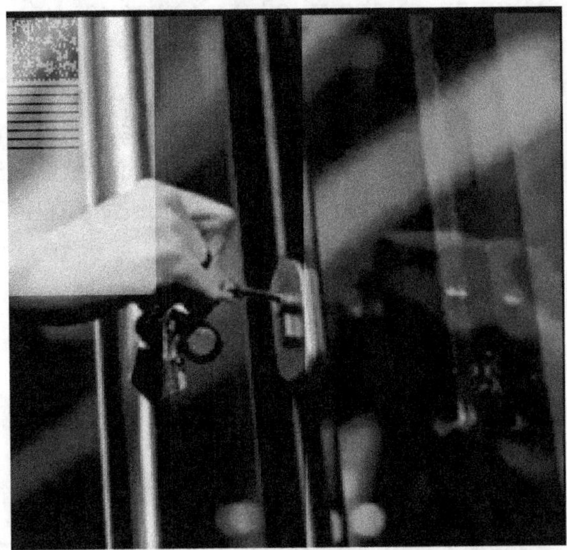

1.   FORMATION/MAKING:

To make simply means *to create, construct, or produce*. Formation simply means something possessing structure or form (the shape or visible structure of a thing or person), this implies that a woman has been in existence but not visible because she has been inside of a man and is this process of formation that makes her visible.

Have you ever wondered why when God discovered that it is not good that the man should be alone (that's both the male man and the female man inside the male man) in Gen. 2:18, He started forming every beast and living creature of the field and every bird of the air and brought them to Adam in Gen. 2:19? God wanted to find out if Adam will recognize that invisible him when made visible.

It is in the secret place that a woman discovers how she was formed and every detail of that formation. When you discover the materials, you were being formed with, it will go a long way in helping you to know how to handle such a product. Most products are so delicate that the manufacturer always boldly writes on the packaging material that it should be handled with care. The reason is that when mishandled, the product will be destroyed and the aim of manufacturing such product will not be achieved.

Most young ladies are drifting away from the manufacturer original plan, simply because they don't want to dwell with their manufacturer in the secret place to find out how the formation process took place, to know the parts that should be handled with care and the part that should just be handled casually.

2.   INTIMACY/KOINONIA:

Intimacy simply means *feeling, or atmosphere of closeness and openness towards someone else, not necessarily involving sexuality.* It is an atmosphere of oneness, communion, and unbroken fellowship.

Have you ever wondered why God has to put Adam to sleep before forming a woman? Have you ever wondered why God never mind if Adam was awake or not when He was forming the animals of the field and the birds of the air? God needed an unbroken fellowship with the woman, that oneness, that brooding so that the woman will be a reflection of God when she comes out.

The reason why no account was given about the formation of the woman in the bible is that the process was carried out in a secret place and is only been discovered in that atmosphere of openness where deep calls unto deep.

Studies have shown that whatsoever we occupy ourselves

with, we become that thing; consciously and subconsciously. You cannot spend more than 50% of your life in a beer parlor and expect to be something less of a drunkard. He who works with the wise also becomes wise, but when you pitch your tent among fools, you also become one.

Whenever you dwell with God in the secret place, He cast a reflection of Himself upon you, because as you behold Him, you will be transformed from one level of glory to another. Under that atmosphere of intimacy, secrets are shared freely. When you are so intimate with someone, most times you may not even realize that you have a need and the need will be solved. We are so much in need of many things today because we have refused to sustain that intimacy till our needs are being solved without our prior knowledge of those needs. We are so much in a hurry to catch up with what God has not concluded, simply because we think we can do it by ourselves. Or probably faster than God.

Whenever we concentrate on building that intimacy, rather than rushing in and out of the secret place, the result is usually exceedingly great. It is just like going to someone to beg for a certain thing, the person if generous enough will give you just that which you ask of him/her. But, when you concentrate on building a friendship with the person, you receive even when you haven't requested and the good thing about building this friendship and intimacy is that you receive more than you asked for; whenever you ask.

3.   PURPOSE DISCOVERY:

Purpose simply means *a result that is desired; an intention, the reason for which something is done, or the reason is done in a particular way.* According to Myles Munroe *"Purpose is the original intention of the manufacturer."*

The purpose is being discovered and not created, to discover is to remove the cover from; to uncover, to reveal. Everything that God created, is for a purpose and one can only discover one's purpose of existence from the creator or manufacturer.

It is possible to live and die without discovering your purpose and is more disastrous than death itself. You can take for instance that God has carefully formed you in a particular way for you to achieve a particular agenda, and you spend 80 or even 90 years here on earth without knowing what the thing is, let alone attempting to fulfill it. It is a huge waste of heavenly resources, and the worst of it all is that you will give an account of it.

The secret place is where the purpose is being discovered because there is openness. And in that atmosphere of openness, deep secrets are unveiled, age-long secrets are been unveiled.

Have you ever wondered why God choose to take only one rib out of the twelve pairs of ribs?

> **It is 100% possible to live and die without discovering one's purpose, and it is even more disastrous than death in itself.**

It is when the purpose is not being discovered that people live and yet don't have any reason to live but only hope on what the day brings. It is when the purpose is not discovered that inferiority complex sets in, I remember growing up with an inferiority complex, I never thought I am worth achieving anything good, I thought I was inferior to all my mates, friends, in fact, everybody. But when I discovered that God has embedded something in me that my generation awaits, that I was not one freak moving around waiting for people's approval, or one biological accident. I discovered that God carefully knighted me the way I am because of the purpose for which He created me to fulfill, that was when I stopped trying to be everyone else but me.

In our generation today, it is quite so unfortunate that most people have left God's original intention for their lives trying to be every other person but whom God wants them to be. As long as all you desire is to be like someone else, no matter how good you may be at that, you can only become the second best of that person. You cannot even be fulfilled in life because that real you that is been suppressed is crying out for expression. And what you would have done effortlessly; if you are on your track, you find it hard doing, because you are not on your track. You are only trying to go against gravity and therefore need more energy to do that.

Most ladies today are looking for shortcuts, everyone wants to follow the trend. No one wants to pay the price of discovering a new path, trendsetters are no longer found. Mrs. A wants to do what Mrs. B is doing, Mrs. B wants to do what Miss C is doing, and the cycle continues. This just reminds me of some student script that my Mom marks, some students copy to the extent that they even copy the person's name, this is what we are into it now, and we copy to the extent that no single trace of our original self is found again. The rate of imitations and fake is now so rampant that mere writing original on a product does not guarantee its originality.

What is the essence of copying when you can easily discover it? There is always this fulfillment that comes with doing that which you are wired to do. It is the confidence that you have in the manufacturer that makes you trust the product. Most times, people sit so comfortably on a chair simply because they have confidence in the manufacturer. It is this confidence that you have in the producer that builds up your confidence. When we refuse to pay the price of discovering, we suffer an inferiority complex. This is because you have not built up that confidence which only comes from the knowledge of the product from the producer.

> **When we refuse to pay the price of discovering, we suffer an inferiority complex.**

As a woman, you not only need to discover your purpose in the secret place, but you also need to discover that of your children. The early you discover your purpose, the easier it is for you to know whom to marry, the seeds you carry, and every other that pertains to life. This is because when you discover your purpose, you will understand that it is not every man that asks for your hand in marriage that you will marry. You need to find out whether the man's purpose complements yours, you need to find out whether he has that ability to grow with you, or is he someone that will kill your dream and purpose.

The worst that can happen to any woman is to enter marriage without discovering purpose. The disaster is that when you finally discover your purpose, you will alongside discover that you have made the wrong choice. And the sad news is that your destiny and even that of your children may be jeopardized.

Most parents today, have forced their children into doing something that does not enable them to fulfill their purpose, simply because they have refused to pay the price of purpose discovering. Have you bordered to find out God's unique plan for each of your children? Or do you just assume that God has the same plan for all of them simply because they are your children? Not so!

4.   WHOLENESS:

Most ladies today enter marriage hoping to be complete which has led to so many broken homes today. **It is important to note that marriage never makes a woman complete and will never do tomorrow.** God only promised Adam a helper meet that is complementary for him and never the one that will complete him or the one that he will complete because their completeness can only be found in the Creator and not in the creatures. Most young ladies today enter marriages with voids hoping to fill them in their marriages and when such voids are not filled, the marriage will be devoid of happiness and subsequently add to the number of broken homes in the society. The reason is that they seek in humans what only God can provide. It only takes a whole woman to marry a whole man, because when God said in *Gen. 2:24* that the two shall be joined to become one flesh, He never said the halves shall be joined to become one flesh. The uniqueness comes from the whole two being made one, it was never a synergistic reaction whereby one plus one, will give you two. It is the coming together of two whole being that the sovereignty of God is being revealed, it shows us the type of bond that exists between the Holy Trinity, where God the Father, God the Son, and God the Holy Spirit, came together to become one.

> **The uniqueness comes from the whole two being made one, it was never a synergistic reaction whereby one plus one, will give you two.**

It was when Eve was made whole in the secret place that God paraded her before Adam. The reason why most ladies today enter into marriage seeking completeness is that they have refused to remain in the secret place to be made whole in the secret place. It is even funny that most ladies are now helping God to parade themselves as half-baked ladies or unbaked ladies and the danger is that since God is Alpha, He is also Omega and will never finish what He never started.

It is only when these whole two accept to be one that submission becomes easier; most women find it hard to submit to their spouse because they were never made whole before being joined together. No matter how you look at it, as long as the woman is not whole, joining both can never produce one. That is why insecurity, fear, uncertainty… enter most marriages.

5.   TRANSFORMATION:

It is in the secret place that God himself transforms our weakness into strength. It was in the secret place that women like Ester gained the courage to fulfill their purpose of existence.

It is in that secret place that the inferiority complex is being transformed into high self-esteem.

Who knew that this woman of Samaria that can even be

referred to as an adulteress of her time can be transformed into a powerful Evangelist that also created a means for the transformation of many people in her city? *John 4:17-18 (The woman answered him, "I have no husband." Jesus said to her, 'you are right in saying, "I have no husband'; for you had five husbands, and the one you have now is not your husband. What you said is true!"); 4:28-29 (Then the woman left her water jar and went back to the city. She said to the people, "Come and see a man who told me everything I have ever done! He cannot be the Messiah, can he?"); 4-39 (Many Samaritans from that city believed in him because of the woman's testimony, "He told me everything I have ever done).*

6.   BROKENNESS:

Never enter the secret place as a superwoman. You are indeed strong, it is true you can do exploits, but whenever it comes to the secret place, the universal password is brokenness. It is this brokenness that binds our love for God, it makes our love for Him stronger that despite the challenges of life, you can remain steadfast in your walk with God. It is this brokenness that quickens Him to dwell with us in that secret place. Little wonder, you never read where the woman said anything when she was being paraded before the man. A heart-to-heart conversation was going on.

Never enter the secret place as a superwoman.

Mary Magdalene was able to enter the secret place in the presence multitude of people around Jesus because of her brokenness. *(Mark 14:3); And being in Bethany at the house Simon the leper, as He sat at the table, a woman came having an alabaster flask of very costly oil of spikenard. Then she broke the flask and poured it on His head.* She has been forgiven much, and this made her love without reservation. She came with her whole heart, she was not even bothered about what the crowd will say, all that mattered to her was how to gain access to the heart of her

Jesus, and people thought she is going insane, but it was not even her concern. She came with all her life savings. Inside her heart, she will be like, you are free to think of whatever you feel like thinking, but if all I have got is Jesus, it is more than enough for me.

Whenever we come to God with a broken heart, He abandons whatever that He is doing and comes to dwell with us. Psalm 51:17 made it clear to us that God does not despise a broken and contrite heart. It does not matter how heavy or thick, or rotten, or dark your iniquities have been, all it just takes for Him to be drawn to you without reservation is your brokenness. Don't be ashamed to cry before Him when you feel like crying, don't be ashamed to roll on the floor when you feel like doing so. Don't even be hindered by what people will say or do, it is heart-to-heart communication, and the wonderful thing about it is that whichever approach you take, the one who sees the heart of all men knows your motive and will never despise you.

> **Whenever you come to God with a broken and contrite heart, He abandons whatever that He is doing and comes to dwell with you.**

Did you not see how Jesus valued what Mary did and even made it compulsory that, whenever the gospel is preached in the world, that singular act of her brokenness will also be told as a memorial to her? This is Jesus Himself giving us an example of how God values our brokenness.

WISDOM TO CARRY AN 'EXTRA' OIL

Five of them were foolish (thoughtless, without forethought) and five were wise (sensible, intelligent, and prudent).
(Matt. 25:2AMP)

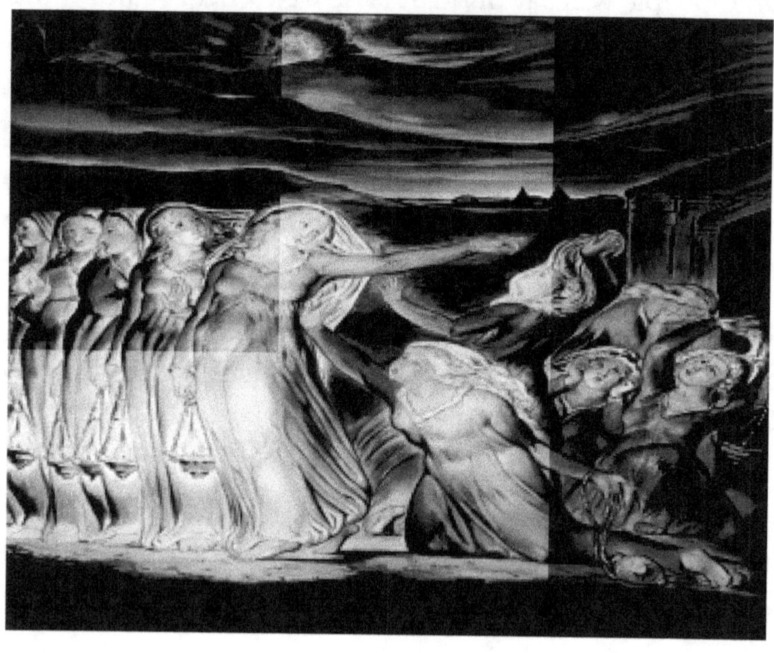

These ten virgins were exposed to the same conditions, they have everything in common; they were all qualified to meet the bridegroom, they had their lamps with oil in them, they were all faced with the challenges of life, they all slept, they all waited, they all persevered, they were even on the alert even as they all slept, they had so many things in common, they were in the same season and time, they weren't even poor!

Why the separation then?

Why then were five referred to as being wise and the other five as foolish?

Why were five of them granted access to the wedding feast, while five were locked outside? Why didn't the bridegroom open the door for them, despite being ready after the door was shut?

Why didn't they leverage on the light from the lamp of the other five wise virgins?

What is the implication of not having extra oil?

LET US TAKE A CLOSER LOOK AT THESE VIRGINS

1. THEY WERE ALL VIRGINS

Wow! These young women were all virgins, oh! I thought this would have been a plus, it's not easy to be a virgin, and it might have cost them a fortune, self-denials, self-disciplines, and other things.

Is being a virgin bad? Not at all. The reason why they were even considered as a case study was that they were virgins. It is this virginity that qualified them to wait for the bridegroom. So, the problem was never their virginity.

So, what then is the problem? Could it be that all they've

got is just this their virginity? Could it be that they became so complacent with this their virginity that they ignorantly refused to work on other areas of their lives? Could it be that they were just living their lives without planning? Could it be that they thought that their virginity could grant them access to all they need in life?

2. THEY TOOK THEIR LAMP

(Matt. 25:1 AMP; *Then the Kingdom of heaven shall be likened to ten virgins who took their lamps and went to meet the bridegroom*).

These young women knew that night may catch up with them on this journey and they took their lamps, why then did the Bible refer to some as being wise and the others foolish?

They were even wise enough to add enough oil in their lamps, why the separation then? Did they make a mistake by carrying their lamp filled with oil for this journey? Oh no, not at all.

They were very successful at the present, very much qualified to meet the bridegroom. Virgins they were, the lamps they had.

3. THEY ALL FELL ASLEEP

What! They all fell asleep, so it was never the sleep. They were all faced with the same human weakness, challenges of life, trials. Why the separation then? They would have all been disqualified if it were all about the limitations of human flesh, but then it was never a criterion because it is generally bound to happen.

Guess what, they all woke up when the alarm was raised about the arrival of the bridegroom. (Matt. 25:6-7 AMP; *But at midnight there was a shout, Behold, the bridegroom! Go out to meet him! Then all those virgins got up and put their lamp in order*).

So, it was never about slumbering or sleeping. These virgins even in their sleep were all vigilant about the coming of the bridegroom, sleep was never a barrier. Even amid their sleep, they all remembered their purpose. They were never ignorant of the fact that they came to meet the bridegroom. It is even unfortunate that most of us today are yet to discover our purpose here on earth, we seem to be occupied with every other thing except that one thing that was in the mind of God when He was forming us.

Have your purpose here on earth entered your subconscious nature that even in your sleep, it is still very gleaming to you? We are in a time where most women are carried away with many things, purpose distractors are everywhere and most women have fallen prey to them. It takes a re-alignment with the Creator to understand the real purpose of our existence here on earth and to likewise work in it.

THE SEPARATION

We have come to a consensus that it was not the carrying of lamp that brought about the separation, neither was it the other five being more virgin than the other five nor was it the delay in the coming of the bridegroom, because they were already referred to as being foolish even before the coming of the bridegroom, which implies that the delay in the coming of the bridegroom was just a revelation/demonstration of their foolishness. It was also not in their falling asleep, because they all fell asleep, it was not even that their lamps were faulty; (Matt. 25:7 AMP; *Then all those virgins got up and put their lamps in order*), and should I shock you a bit, finance was not even the problem because they never borrowed money to go and buy (Matt. 25:9 AMP; *But the wise replied, There will not be enough for us and you; go instead to the dealers and for yourselves*). Their foolishness was never a result of lack of finance nor dealers because they were available even at midnight.

You know taking a close look at these five wise virgins, ignorant people would have said that they were selfish but, the truth is that when you fail to plan your life, you should not be envious of those who have done so, or accuse them of not showing empathy.

Note that it is not all the time that life will afford you the opportunity of covering your foolishness, even if it does most times, would you rather live your life on what the day brings? It is not all the time that you can borrow things to cover up for your inabilities. Neither is it all the time that you have the opportunity of leveraging on other peoples' success.

This calls for wisdom! What was lacking in the lives of these young virgins were wisdom, foresight, and lack of proper planning, like the general saying that he who fails to plan, plans to fail. You see, even when you refuse to plan, life has a way of planning for you, but the bad news is that it is to fail. Is that the plan you have for your life? Would you rather allow life to do the planning when God has wired in you all it takes to have the foresight and take part in the revelation of His wisdom?

> **It was never lack of finance that made the foolish virgins not carry extra oil, it was lack of wisdom, foresight, and proper planning.**

Since these five virgins were able to buy the oil, they were still not granted access to the marriage feast and were termed unprepared. What! I thought the oil is the cause of the separation, oh! The bridegroom must have been so unfair not to have allowed them in, look these virgins are ready with their extra oil and yet we're not allowed into the marriage feast. So, what then is the problem? Is the bridegroom unjust? Certainly NO, the timing of the readiness was the problem. (Matt. 25:10 AMP; *But while they were going away to buy, the bridegroom came, and **those who were prepared** went in with him to the marriage feast, **and the door was shut**).* The issue now is no longer those who have extra oil but those who were prepared at that particular point in time; at that particular point in time, the door was open for all the ten virgins to enter, but there were at the wrong place at the right time.

What if you are ready but on a shut door? I remember vividly how I prepaid for an 8 am lecture on Friday 14th May 2021. I was directly facing the door, with some of my colleagues when the Lecturer shut the door at exactly 8 am. Was I prepared for the class? 100% prepared. Was I granted access to the lecture? 0%.

So, it's not all about the preparation. Yes, it is not an easy thing to prepare for something, but the timing of the preparation is as crucial as the preparation itself; if not more crucial than the preparation itself.

You can imagine preparing a beautiful wedding cake a day after the wedding, no matter how beautiful the cake is, it is useless for the occasion. Not necessarily because it is not well prepared, but because it was ready at the wrong time.

What if you are at the right place at the wrong time? The next chapter will reveal the implications of being ready at the wrong time.

> **The problem is not with being prepared, but the timing of the readiness.**

This time of being ready is very important because being ready at the wrong time is as bad as not preparing at all. The popular saying that, "it is better late than never" does not apply here. Sometimes being late is worse than not preparing at all.

THE CONCEPT 'TIME'

***Later** the **other virgins** also came and said, Lord, Lord, open [the door] to us!*

(Matt. 25:11 AMP)

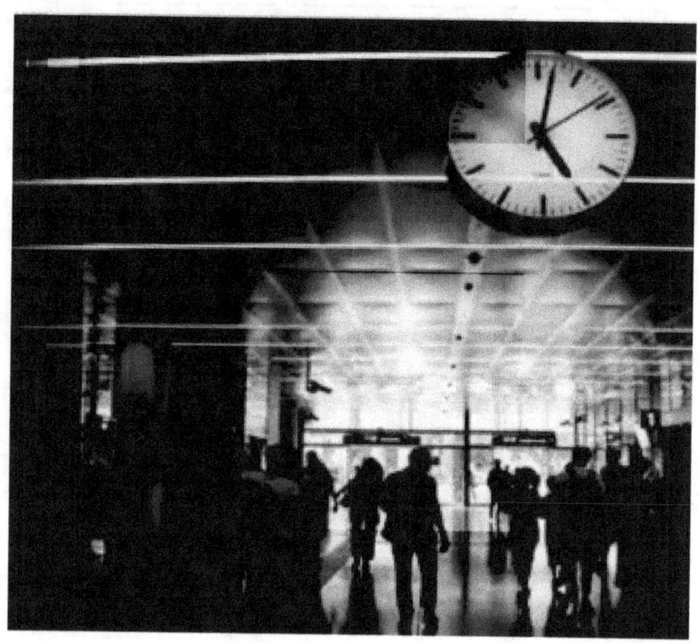

The word 'Concept' simply means an understanding retained in the mind, from experience, reasoning, and/ or imagination; a generalization, or abstraction, of a particular set of instances or occurrences. While the word 'TIME'

simply means: The inevitable progression into the future with the passing of present events into the past. The particular moment or hour; the appropriate moment or hour for something. To choose when something begins or how long it lasts.

These five foolish virgins were ready to meet the bridegroom now with the extra oil that was the reason why they were referred to as being foolish, but then the door was shut.

The Bible made it so clear that they were no longer foolish virgins but 'other virgins,' but that still did not remove the fact that they were held back by a shut door. There is something remarkable about these other virgins, they never give up on their dreams, they bought the oil, came back to meet the bridegroom, they were optimistic, but despite all these, they were all happening at the 'later,' at the wrong time. They were all happening at the inappropriate moment or hour for the feast. Loo and behold the reply of the bridegroom *I solemnly declare to you; I do not know you [I am not acquainted with you]* (Matt. 25:12).

Had there been no time in this equation, these ten virgins are just qualified to meet the bridegroom face to face! Had they had an understanding of the time and season; they would have been inside the marriage feast. One thing is certain and that is the fact that **there is a marriage feast;** despite the delay, **the bridegroom will certainly come,** there will be a shout, **and only those who are prepared and present at the moment, will go into the marriage feast with the bridegroom and** Lastly, **the door will be shut to separate those who are prepared AT THAT PARTICULAR MOMENT, from those who are not.**

One peculiar thing about our ephemeral life is that we are time-bound. Everything that we do revolves around time, and whoever fails to manage/maximize his/her time, leads to a result that is usually disastrous.

"While the earth remains, seedtime and harvest, cold and heat, winter and summer, and day and night shall not cease." (Gen. 8:22). As long as we are on this planet Earth, times and seasons will always persist. If we know that something is certain, the best we can do for ourselves is to maximize it. And how can you maximize

what you do not understand?

Ecclesiastes 3:1 made it clear to us that there is a season for everything and a time for every purpose under heaven. Woe betide you if you do not understand the time for your purpose here on earth!

Not understanding the time for a particular purpose is like putting on a thick cardigan during the summer season and expecting a harvest when you have not done what you are meant to do during the seedtime. It is foolishness to expect a harvest when you have not sowed and the worst of it all is for you to consume or waste your seed. Proverbs 24:33 made it clear to us that a **little** sleep, a **little** slumber, and a **little** folding of the hands to rest, is an open invitation to poverty.

It is foolishness to sleep away your working hours! And the dangerous aspect of it is that it happens gradually and even unnoticed. You might just be thinking that it's just a little, and won't have any effect. But that is a lie. If you have been sleeping 8 hours a day, that means that in 10 years, you have slept for 29,200 hours just in 10 years and that will not prevent you from sleeping today. It is time for us to wake up from our slumber, time to spread out those folded hands and maximize every single time.

The fact that you refused to do what you are supposed to do, does not mean that your needs will refuse to come. Proverbs 24:34 made it clear that the needs will come like an armed man and one thing with armed men is that nobody anticipates them, and whenever they come, you must always give them what they are asking for.

Proper understanding of times and seasons help us to maximize our destiny and purpose here on earth. The Bible talked about the sons of Issachar in 1 Chronicle 12:32 as those that had an understanding of the times, they were very little compared to other tribes, but they had a very distinct quality which was their ability to understand the times. The good thing with the understanding of times is that it gives you leverage over others and you always know what to do at every given season. The Bible made it clear that they knew what Israel ought to do.

> **Proper understanding of times and seasons help us to maximize our destiny and purpose here on earth.**

Most ladies are so confused about what to do at every season of their lives simply because they have failed to understand the times. Some don't even know when the change and that automatically renders them incapacitated. Times and seasons go hand in hand, and when you lack understanding of the current time, you will most likely miss out on what is expected of the season.

Most business organizations have gone into extinction today simply because they failed to understand that times have changed and instead of upgrading, they remained where they were, and finally, they go into extinction. That is how it is for most ladies today, they fail to understand when the seasons of their lives change and don't even know that there is a need to upgrade, and that is how they remain extinct in the new season.

Most ladies keep doing the same thing over and over again expecting different results. It is a sign of immaturity and lack of wisdom to keep doing the same thing over and over again and expect a different result. If simple phone applications need constant upgrading, how much more a woman that is a rational being! Most ladies even find it difficult to let go of the previous season, even when it is very obvious to them that the season has changed.

For growth to occur, you have to let go of some things and embrace the new one; no matter how you have valued them. Even before a grain of wheat produces more grains, it will first fall into the ground and die, if not, it remains just a grain. If you so cherish such a grain of wheat, you may be so protective that you don't even want it to fall into the ground, let alone die.

The truth is that for you to remain relevant in each season, you need to understand the times and do the necessary upgrading which usually alters the status quo.

> **If simple phone applications need constant upgrading, how much more a woman that is a rational being!**

Don't you know that in that marriage you are entering into or already into that trial time is bound to come? Don't you know that the bridegroom could be delayed? Don't you know that the perseverance test would be conducted? What capacity have you built like the woman that you are? What is that which you know that could deliver you and your family from the shackles of the enemy? What is it that can distinguish you from the crowd? What is that extra thing that you have acquired? What is the extra skill, the knowledge that you have acquired, that will make you stand out among equals? Do you want to end up like every other person? Do you want to stop where every other person stopped?

Funny enough, life has a way of revealing all these lapses no matter how you wish to hide them. Have you gained mastery over the times and seasons of your life? Have you acquired the necessary skills and knowledge to keep you relevant in each season of your life? Do you have the foresight and understanding of times of your life to know what to do in every season of your life? Or are you just waiting for what the day brings! Or to remain extinct in the ever-changing times and seasons?

> **For growth to occur, you have to let go of some things and embrace the new one; no matter how you have valued them.**

It is time to be deliberate; intentional about your life and purpose. What makes extraordinary what it is, is not the absence of ordinary, but the addition of that word **'extra.'** The word 'Extra' simply means beyond what is due, usual, expected, or necessary; extraneous; additional; supernumerary... What is that extra thing you are doing that no one else can do? How willing are you, to move an extra mile where others stopped? What extra effort have you put in place to carve a niche for yourself, to stand out among equals?

> **What makes extraordinary what it is, is not the absence of ordinary, but the addition of that word 'extra.'**

There is more to being a woman than just being a woman. **You are not just another man; you are a man with a womb!**

Now, what does this implies? There is more to your being a woman. It is important to find out what this womb has conferred on you, it is important to discover the implication of that womb. It is important to understand that God is not too jobless to have put a womb inside of a man and called that man 'woman' even before Adam did so! We will dwell more on the above in the next chapter.

> **You are not just another man; you are a man with a womb!**

HE MADE ME A WOMAN

And the rib or part of his side which the Lord God had taken from the man He built up and made into a woman, and He brought her to the man.

(Genesis 2:22)

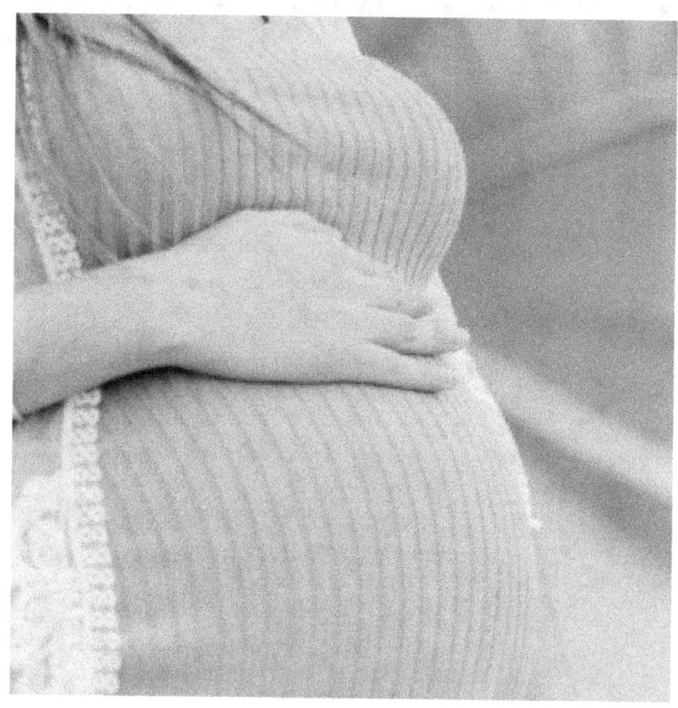

HE BUILT UP AND MADE INTO A WOMAN!

Having looked into what happened to the rib in the secret place, it is important to look into the end product of that building up; a woman.

The building up and making of a woman remains a mystery till today and it is only unveiled to those who are willing to search out that mystery in the secret place. What does it mean to be a woman? Does being a woman just signifies the title given to any human being that is not a man? Not at all. There is more to being a woman, than just answering woman. And we will sequentially look into these qualities of a woman.

If only we could understand what it means to be a woman, we wouldn't have been wasting time struggling for equality. This is because the presence of the womb in a woman has conferred some qualities that can never be found in any man. Isn't it wonderful to know that as a woman, you are not just a man but a man with a womb? It's like saying that as a woman, you are a man plus womb. It can be mathematically represented as Woman = Man + Womb. So, as a woman, you have the attributes of a man, and also the attributes that the womb confers.

God was so meticulous in the making of a woman because He has seen the lapses in the first edition of creation. The first edition of human creation was lacking in the ability to make good and God has to intervene, He gathered all the whole raw materials both in heaven and on earth and entered His inner chamber to build, and made the updated and last edition of creation, His own very last born that is very dear and close to His heart.

Do you not wonder the reason why God had to start forming every beast and living creature of the field and every bird of the air even when He has discovered that it was not good for the man whom He has created in His image and likeness to be alone!

God wanted her to be the last born of His creation. In the process of the building up, He emptied Himself in her.

Have you taken into consideration why the word 'built up' was used, instead of just saying that the rib was made into a woman? It is because the building up involved a process that God Himself didn't want to make open.

It was not just something that happened in minutes or hours, it was a process. God was wiring so many things into this being, to the point that He was fully satisfied and proud of this process of building up and now put the inscription 'woman' on her.

On a normal, He would have just waited for Adam to give the product of the formation its name as He did with the livestock and birds of the air; (*(Genesis 2: 19) And out of the ground the Lord God formed every [wild] beast and living creature of the field and every bird of the air **and brought them to Adam to see what he would call them; and whatever** Adam called every living creature, that was its name*).

God didn't want to do trials and error in this updated and last edition of His creation by just allowing Adam to call her **whatever** name he wishes, rather this one was already called a woman even before bringing her to **the man**; (*(Genesis 2: 22) And the rib or part of his side which the Lord God had taken from the man He built up and made into a woman, and **He brought her to the man**)*. Note, God didn't bring the woman to the man to see what he will call her, because she has already been given a name by her builder. God only paraded her before the man to know if actually, he will recognize that she is a help suitable.

It is important to also note that the woman was brought to the man and not Adam (May God grant you understanding). Most times, we may just casually read the bible and assume that some words are used out of convenience, not at all.

Do you know that God deliberately brought the woman before the man and not Adam? Because He wanted to institute the office of a husband and a wife. He wanted to make it clear to the man that this thing I am about instituting transcends beyond Adam and Eve, that you can be paraded before any man from which you can be married to and not just restricted to Mr. A, or B, that the most important thing is for the man to recognize that you are a help suitable.

> **God didn't bring the woman to the man to see what he will call her, because she has already been called a woman.**

Sometimes, I use to wonder why God had to put Adam to sleep, not just any sleep, but a deep one for that matter. And I came to understand that He wanted to finish the building process, He wanted to build up a creature that can be a true replica of His creative nature, a creature that will be so compassionate as His very self, a creature that will have the ability to nurture.

He was so proud of this last born of His creation that He wanted everything about creation to be concluded before building His end of discussion. He even has to put His logo on her, He wanted maximum concentration, an intimacy that is devoid of every distraction, which is why He has to put the man into a deep sleep.

As a woman, if you are still waiting for a man to let you know that you are a woman, then something is seriously wrong somewhere because it will be a vain waiting. He doesn't even have a glimpse of how you became a woman. What you ought to wait for, is for the man to recognize that you are a help suitable.

> **A woman is the updated and last edition of God's creation.**

Only God knows how long He stayed with the woman before parading her before the man. No wonder women always know the right button to press and God will be moved to come to their rescue, they have stayed so long with God they know His desires. They understand what their tears do to the heart of God and how it moves Him to come to their rescue.

You may be wondering why women always cry, it's not their fault, they are emotional beings and have full knowledge of what each drop of those tears does to the heart of God. The first time Jesus wept in the bible was because He saw a woman crying; *(John 11:33-35) [33] Therefore, **when Jesus saw her weeping,** and the Jews who came with her weeping, He groaned in the spirit and was troubled. [34] And He said, "Where have you laid him?" They said to Him, "Lord, come and see." [35] Jesus wept.*

> **Women always cry because they have full knowledge of what each drop of those tears does to the heart of God.**

It is true that Jesus came to see and bring back Lazarus from death, that God will be glorified, but He was still reluctant about it, it is evidenced in verse 30 of the 11th chapter of John's account of the gospel; *Now Jesus had not yet come into the town, but was in the place where Martha met Him.* You will agree with me that He was reluctant about bringing back to the life of Lazarus, why would He stay back to the point that Martha had to go back to the house, inform Mary of His presence and Mary also had to walk to the place where He was.

Your identity as a woman when fully discovered and maximized, you will be amazed to see the wonders that will come out of it. We will be looking at some of the intrinsic abilities domicile in a woman. When these abilities are known and maximized, it will end competitions and birth forth women that know their worth and women that live out their full potentials here on earth. The earlier we realize what it means to be a woman, the earlier we stop looking for what we are not, and start maximizing that which we are.

IS BEING A WOMAN A DISADVANTAGE?

We are living in a world where things could make someone think that being a woman is a disadvantage. But since this may seem like a fact, it is never the truth. This issue of seeing being a woman as a disadvantage is more prominent or even predominant in African countries.

This has made most women live below what is expected of them. It has led many into inferiority complex syndrome while many are just living as the day brings. Most women have even believed that it is indeed the man world and therefore, they don't offer their best to the world.

Some have been made to believe that they are the weaker vessel, which may still appear to be true, but it is not. Women are not just powerful, but they have authority. This authority, when understood and applied, can produce a tremendous result that cannot be accomplished by 100 men with their assumed stronger vessel.

It will be absolute wastage of time and resources trying to compete with men or struggling for equality because you are subtly superior if only you can maximize all that has been deposited inside of you. The only problem that we have as women, is that we have failed to discover what is inside of us and have resorted to chasing shadows ignoring the real image.

> **Women are not just powerful, but they have authority. This authority, when understood and applied, can produce a tremendous result.**

Being a woman is never a disadvantage and will never be a disadvantage. Being a woman is not just an advantage but a privilege and should be welcomed. You can never gain value from what you despise. You only gain value from what you accept and value. The reason why most women do not gain the value of being a woman, it's because they don't even accept the fact that they are women, let alone value it.

The reason why most females become turn-boy is simply that they don't know why they are female, and instead of discovering why they are female, they resort to turn-boy simply because their environment has propelled them to believe that acting like a male is the main thing, while being a female that they are in the secondary thing.

This problem of most females not understanding whom they are do not just start with them, it is an error that started from their mothers and is being passed unto them. It, therefore, requires immediate intervention. The reason is simple, and it is that you cannot give what you don't have. When we fail to discover who we are as women, it does not just end with us but, it is been passed unto our children and the cycle continues until someone pays that price of discovery.

The annoying aspect of this lack of self-discovery by the mothers is that their daughters may even ask them some sensitive questions about themselves and they cannot provide the answer. And of course, it is not surprising since one cannot give what the person doesn't have. We have passed the days of ignorance and this is time for women to discover who they are and break this cycle of lack of knowledge, apply the acquired understanding in their lives and that of their children, and society at large, to make the world a better place for themselves and that of their society at large.

> **This problem of most women not understanding whom they do not just start with them, it is an error that started from their mothers and is being passed unto them.**

The bible made us understand in Psalms 139:14 that we are fearfully and wonderfully made, why then do we want to deviate from this His wonderfully made plan just to follow the trend, and end up not being who He made us be? The danger here is that there is no divine provision outside what God has purposed.

The birds can fly because God has built-in flying abilities in them, the fishes can swim because God has built-in swimming abilities in them. If the fish all of a sudden decide to fly, despite how much hard it tries, it can never do it like the birds, if at all it can do it. Likewise, if the bird suddenly decides to swim instead of flying, no matter how hard it tries, it can never swim better than the fish if at all it can swim. And the reason is not far-fetched, God did not put the ability to swim inside of the bird, neither did he put the ability to fly inside of the fishes.

> **We have passed the days of ignorance and this is time for women to discover who they are and break this cycle of lack of knowledge, apply the acquired understanding in their lives and that of their children, and society at large.**

We as women, no matter how hard we try to be a turn-boy or turn-man, can never be as effective as the man. And the reason is also not far-fetched, there is a womb inside of the man in us, which has added some qualities in us that can never be found in men. And this implies that no matter how hard a woman tries to be a man, she can never be a man as effective as the man himself, and that is if it is even possible for her to be just a man.

What is now the need of trying to be someone else, when you

can maximize who you are made to be? What is now the reason for mimicking or imitating when there is room for the original? What is now the reason for being a first runner up, when you can become the winner? What is now the reason for living below standard when you have access to the standard? What is now the reason for trying to be a half-baked woman, when the baker has not switch-off the ovum? What is now the reason for staggering when you have access to light? What is the reason for visiting the place of your unveiling when you have been given an invitation to dwell? What is the reason for the lack of understanding when the knowledge can be accessed? What is the reason for trying to copy when the scroll has been given to you as a possession? What is the reason for not being a woman God has made you be when he has embedded all it takes to be a woman inside of you?

This is time for us to stop looking around for a while and look within, to discover that which has been freely given to us for being a woman, and maximize it to the fullness. This is time to go back to the drawing board to discover where there is a missing link and then bridge the gap. This is time for us to go back to that ancient pathway to discover where we have missed the path in-order to bridge that path because no matter how hard you try to cover up without going back to the origin of the problem to solve the problem from there, the lapses will always show up.

Let us now stop treating the symptoms of the illness, ignoring the illness. Since treating the symptoms does not eliminate the illness but only grant a momentary relief and keeps on reoccurring. The earlier we take the bull by the horn and stop these trials and errors with our identity as a woman, the better for us. The earlier we stop struggling for shadows and concentrate on the real image, the better for us.

When we consider our being a woman as a disadvantage, we can never maximize all that we have for being a woman. The truth is that it is never a disadvantage to be a woman, and can never be a disadvantage. There is more to being a woman than just being a woman, and when this more is being tapped into and maximized, it produces a tremendous result that leaves the world in awe.

> **This is time for us to stop looking around for a while and look within, to discover that which has been freely given to us for being a woman and maximize it to the fullness.**

The danger of not discovering and appreciating who you are as the woman that you are, it's that other people are doing so. Therefore, don't think that because you have failed to pay the price of discovering, that others are just folding their hands like you. So, brace up and do the needful when there is still time, for a time cometh when it will be too late to apply that knowledge.

INTRINSIC ABILITIES IN WOMAN

If God has ever been so deliberate in His creative work, then the woman is the product of that scientific and artwork of God. He was so intentional in the making of a woman, He has seen all the lapses in the first edition of man and now gathered all the whole heavenly, humanly and Godly resources to make and build up His end of discussion.

After the building up and the making of a woman, you never heard anything about creation from God. Do you know why? He has intrinsically embedded all it takes to procreate inside of a woman. He was so meticulous in building up her physiological organs to achieve all His aim of creating her.

If you listened very closely when God finished the building up and making of a woman, you will hear Him say it is finished. And the reason why He may say such is that He has embedded in her all that is needed to continue His creative work, all that is needed to make good of the man He has created, all that is needed to make good of the family He has instituted, all that is needed to make good of the society, all that is needed to make good of mankind, and all that is needed to make good of all He has created.

> **After the building up and making of a woman, you never heard anything about creating again, because**

> **God has embedded all it takes to procreate inside of her.**

We will be taking a closer look at some of these intrinsic abilities that God has meticulously wired inside of this creature called woman. An understanding of these abilities will help the woman to appreciate her nature and also maximize these God-given abilities to the glory of His name. It is very crucial that every woman understand these intrinsic abilities, because when you lack knowledge and understanding of what you have, it does not negate the fact that it's in you, but it jeopardizes its purpose of being inherent in you. And the bad effect of it is that you tend to abuse such purpose, and this was never the original intention of God concerning those abilities.

The next chapters will be unveiling to us some of the intrinsic abilities embedded in a woman, how they can be maximized to make good of the man, family, and society at large. When women understand these intrinsic abilities and apply them through the help of their maker, the world will be a better place to live in.

EMBEDDED IN EVERY WOMAN, IS THE INTRINSIC ABILITY TO MAKE GOOD

*(Gen. 2:18; Now the Lord God said, it is **not good** (sufficient, satisfactory) that the man should be alone; I **will** make him a **helper meet** (suitable, adapted, complementary) for him.)*

As long as you are a woman, you don't need to struggle to make good, because it's already inherent in you! If you are struggling to make good, then there is a knowledge gap that needs to be filled. Because God has wired the ability to make good in you, as long as you accept to be a woman.

I used the word accept to be a woman because most people seriously find it had to accept that they are women, that is why some tend to become turn-boy or the likes. The resources only become available when you truly accept to be a woman. And that is because you attract what you accept.

Your making good has a lot to do with the man you choose to submit to as a husband. If you choose a man who doesn't see the good in you, your ability to make good, will be adulterated. If you choose a man who sees everything good in every woman but you, who end up comparing you with other women, your ability to make good, will be dysfunctional even though it has been wired to be functional. This is because in every man lies the intrinsic ability to do the vice, and being a woman doesn't deny the fact that you are also a man, but with a womb as well. So, when you become a helpmeet to a man whom you are not compatible with, your ability to make good, will be adulterated, even though it's in you, and that is because you cannot force a square peg into a round hole.

> **As long as you are a woman, you don't need to struggle to make good, because it's already inherent in you.**

That's why it is a very wise decision to choose wisely when it comes to choosing a life partner. Because it goes a long way to affect your ability to make good, the quality of the help suitable you will become. That was why God didn't bring the woman to Adam, but the man so that you won't be restricted in your decision-making.

You can agree with me that if the man didn't recognize that the woman is a help suitable, God would have paraded the woman to another man. Do you know why? The building-up process was well concluded before bringing the woman out to the man and the ability to make good was well wired in her.

This intrinsic ability of the woman to make good goes beyond that of the man, it cuts across the whole society, the children, and the family. Any woman who truly understands what being a woman calls for, makes good of anything that comes her way.

With a proper support system, the woman can maximize all that has been intrinsically embedded in her to make good. You won't say that because she can make good that when subjected to any condition that she can do it.

Most women who grew in an abusive home, hardly emerge as perfect good-maker, simply because the environment they found themselves in didn't support their growth. No matter how good the seed maybe, when planted in poor soil it tends to have stunted growth which invariably affects the future seeds. This is why the growth of every woman should be handled with care because whenever there is a default in her ability to make good, it goes beyond her to affect her next generation, society, husband, family, and everyone connected to her.

> **With a proper support system, the woman can maximize all that has been intrinsically embedded in her to make good.**

Any wise man who wants to produce a tremendous result out of his dream can communicate such a dream to the woman and no matter how bad it may be, the intrinsic ability of the woman to make good will always make it good. Any woman who has truly understood this her intrinsic ability to make good can make good of every situation irrespective of how bad the situation might have been.

> **Any woman who has truly understood this her intrinsic ability to make good can make of every situation irrespective of how bad the situation might have been.**

EMBEDDED IN EVERY WOMAN, IS THE INTRINSIC ABILITY TO INFLUENCE

I love the Merriam-Webster definition of influence and it states "the power to change or affect someone or something. The power to cause changes without directly forcing them to happen."

Any woman, no matter the age or size has the intrinsic ability to influence any man despite his age. The beautiful thing about this influential power of a woman is that it is done without directly forcing them to happen.

1. **The first miracle performed by Jesus was as a result of the influential power of a woman;**

(John 2: 3 – 5) [3] And when they ran out of wine, the mother of Jesus said to Him, "They have no wine." [4] Jesus said to her, "Woman, what does your concern have to do with me? My hour has not yet come." [5] His mother said to the servants, "Whatever He says to you, do it."

Jesus had no plan of performing any miracle He was even wondering why the mother was so concerned about what does not concern them, but because of the intrinsic ability of women to influence, He later performed the miracle even against His timing. And the most interesting aspect of it is the fact that the mother was able to influence Him without directly forcing Him.

The mother of Jesus understood perfectly the influential power of women, she didn't even bother convincing Him or start explaining to Him why she is concerned about the fact that they don't have wine, she just used the influential power of women and went to the servants.

You will agree with me that she also used this influential power on the servants! See, Jesus has never performed any miracle before them, they were acting under the influence of a woman; *"Whatever He says to you, do it."* It is only this influence that can make a full-fleshed man obey such instructions as these; *(John 2:7-8)*

[7] Jesus said to them, "Fill the waterpots with water." And they filled them up to the brim.

[8] And He said to them, "Draw some out now, and take it to the master of the feast." And they took it.

This is something that has never happened before, they didn't even consider the implications of what they were doing. Can you imagine! The instruction was not even to give it to one of them or to even Jesus himself but to the master of the feast. Their ego was at stake, their achievements and how people will see them, was even at stake. You can imagine how the master of the feast would have used the microphone to disgrace them before the crowd, but they didn't consider all these things because they have been influenced by a woman.

You may be thinking that they didn't act under the influence of a woman, but look at what happened thereafter; *(John 2:9-11)*

[9] When the master of the feast had tasted the water that was made wine, and did not know where it came from (but the servants who had drawn the water knew), the master of the feast called the bridegroom.

[10] And he said to him, "Every man at the beginning sets out the good wine, and when the guests have well drunk, then the inferior. You have kept the good wine until now!" [11] This beginning of signs Jesus

did in Cana of Galilee and manifested His glory, and His disciples believed in Him).

> **Any woman, no matter the age or size have the intrinsic ability to influence any man; despite his age**

Note that, it was after the miracle happened that the disciples believed in Him. So now, what do you think made them carry out such an unprecedented instruction? It is simply the influential power of a woman. Never underestimate what the influential power of a woman can make a man do.

2. The Jews were saved from the king's decree because of the influence of a woman:
(Esther 5:1-3)
[1] Now it happened on the third day that Esther put on her royal robes and stood in the inner court of the king's palace, across from the king's house, while the king sat on his royal throne in the royal house, facing the entrance of the house.
[2] So it was when the king saw Queen Esther standing in the court that she found favor in his sight, and the king held out to Esther the golden scepter that was in his hand. Then Esther went near and touched the top of the scepter.
[3] And the king said to her, "What do you wish, Queen Esther? What is your request? It shall be given to you—up to half the kingdom!"

Queen Esther used the influence of a woman to deliver the Jewish people from the king's decree that would have brought about their end. She did it in such a way that the king was even in a hurry to obey her wish. The steps were meticulously calculated and it yielded the expected result.

Whenever a woman puts on her whole regalia of womanhood, nothing is unachievable for her. All it takes is just for her to understand that this power is inherent in her, and with this full understanding, she can make anyone dance to her tune.

Little wonder the King was not even concerned about the fact that she has violated the king's law, all he was concerned about was what she wished for.

> **Whenever a woman puts on her whole regalia of womanhood, nothing is unachievable for her.**

Queen Esther has not even mentioned her petitions and because of the influence, he couldn't sleep. *(Esther 6:1) That night the king could not sleep. So, one was commanded to bring the book of the records of the chronicles; and they were read before the king.* He was already restless, wondering what the request could be. What could have made a king promise to do whatever the request could be, even up to half the kingdom?

3. The first time Jesus revealed his identity as the Christ was before a woman:
(John 4:25-26)
[25] The woman said to Him, "I know that Messiah is coming" (who *is called Christ). "When He comes, He will tell us all things."*
*[26] Jesus said to her, "**I who speak to you am He.**"*

There is something very remarkable about women, Jesus just told this woman that He is the Christ, while He has not made mention of that before; even to His disciples. I can imagine how happy He was talking with this woman and the look in the face of His disciples when they came back. ((*John 4:27 And at this point His disciples came, and they marveled that He talked with a woman; yet no one said, "What do You seek?" or, "Why are You talking with her?"*). What! Is our master about to marry, this and many more will be going on in their minds.

The Samaritan woman, was able to influence men in her city;
(John 4:28-30)
*[28] The woman then left her waterpot, went her way into the city, **and said to the men,***
*[29] "Come, see a Man who told me all things that I ever did. **Could this be the Christ?**"*

[30] Then they went out of the city and came to Him.

Note this woman didn't even spend any time convincing them, as a matter of fact, she just asked them a question and they all left what they were doing to follow her.

Don't be deceived into thinking that women are easily deceived, it may look like the truth, but may not be true. And the truth is that even though men claim not to be easily deceived, they are easily influenced by a woman.

This woman in question has a questionable reputation, yet she still influences the men. *((John 4:39) And many of the Samaritans of that city believed in Him because of the word of the woman who testified, "He told me all that I ever did.")*

Never allow the devil to deceive you into believing that your inherent ability to influence will be removed because you have sinned in the past, as long as you have truly asked for forgiveness, there is no condemnation for you and God's given abilities in you remains in you. It will be a waste of resources of heaven if after investing so much in you, your refuse to maximize those abilities because of ignorance. But this ability was placed inside of us by God, and the original plan of it is for it to be used for a good purpose and never the other way around

The list could go on and on, the Bible is filled with so many scenarios where the influential power of women were been displayed. The Israelites were delivered from the hand of the Sisera in Judges Chapter 4 because of the influence of a woman; *(Judges 4:8-9) [8] And Barak said to her, If you will go with me, then I will go; but if you will not go with me, I will not go.*

*[9] And she said, I will surely go with you; nevertheless, the trip you take will not be for your glory, **for the Lord will sell Sisera into the hand of a woman**. And Deborah arose and went with Barak to Kedesh. [Fulfilled in Judg. 4:22.]*

John the Baptist, the forerunner of Jesus Christ was beheaded, just because of the influence of a woman (see Matthew 14:3-10).

Looking at Adam and Eve in the garden of Eden, the devil was able to entice the woman, because she loves hearing sweet things; she's easily moved by what she hears and is also attracted to beautiful things; *(Genesis 3:4-6)*

[4] Then the serpent said to the woman, "You will not surely die.

[5] For God knows that in the day you eat of it your eyes will be opened, and you will be like God, knowing good and evil."

*[6] So when the woman saw that the tree was good for food, that it was pleasant to the eyes, and a tree desirable to make one wise, she took of its fruit and ate. **She also gave to her husband with her**, and he ate.*

She has already calculated all the benefits that they will get by eating the fruit and what they were scared of before, which is that they will die, she has been informed that she won't die, so she decided to explore not knowing that the devil has been a liar from the very beginning. The devil understood this influential power of the woman that is why he didn't bother saying anything to Adam. Because he knew that if he succeeds in altering the mindset of the woman that she can easily influence the husband.

Every woman needs to have access to full knowledge of whom they are as a woman, they need to understand their position because whatever gains access through the woman into the family, it will gain access into every other member of the family. That is why the man needs to be a covering to them. It's only a foolish man that pushes the wife to the forefront of destruction, because anything that permeates her, will effortlessly permeate every other member of the family.

It is because most women don't understand what it takes to be a woman that they live their life so casually, allowing whatever flies around to gain access into their lives. And the bad effect of it is that if God did not intervene, it passes over to their children and the cycle continues.

EMBEDDED IN EVERY WOMAN, IS THE ABILITY TO BE A SEED CARRIER

Women by default are seed carriers, and that is a God-given ability in them. God has meticulously wired this ability in women and that is why seeds don't die in their hands. The ability to be a seed carrier is part of what the womb by physiology conferred on women.

No matter how strong a man claims to be, he lacks that intrinsic ability to be a seed carrier. This women's ability to be a seed carrier goes beyond just being pregnant for nine months and giving birth to a child, it cuts across the man's visions, dreams, purpose, ambition, careers, vocations, and every other thing that can be birthed forth.

> **No matter how strong a man claims to be, he lacks that intrinsic ability to be a seed carrier.**

Women are seed carriers and not seed givers, that is why they are just neutral about the gender of their children and this neutral nature is evidenced in the way she loves each one equally.

Every human being, and even most other mammals have two sex chromosomes; the X chromosome which is responsible for the female gender when in pairs (XX); one from the man and one from the woman, and the Y chromosome, which is responsible for male gender when combined with one of the X chromosomes from the woman to give XY chromosomes. The woman has two X chromosomes, while the man has both X and Y chromosomes, and whichever one he gives the woman, who is naturally a receiver, she carries and brings forth.

It baffles me how some men, especially in the African continent divorce their wife simply because she couldn't give birth to a particular gender, not knowing that it was a garbage-in, garbage out process and that the woman does not determine the sex of her child. God in His infinite wisdom has designed it to be so. He knows that such a time will come when the gender of the child will be questioned, and because He loves taking sides with the women, he just prevented them from such impending trouble.

Now, looking at this ability to be a seed carrier, the woman undergoes so many physiological, psychological, and hormonal changes and adaptations to carry and bring forth its seed. These nine months of pregnancy is never an easy one, it is a battle between survival and death, why because another life is coming forth. The appetites of the woman change, she has to accommodate the seed, most times she requests for something unimaginable, something that on a normal she will detest, just to accommodate the seed she is carrying. She becomes a co-life giver with God because she has been wired to do so.

That is why any man that understands this intrinsic ability of the woman to be a seed carrier, always trusts her with his vision and purpose, knowing full well that the vision will not die in her hand. She will deny herself so many things just to accommodate that vision, she can even deprive herself of comfort, just to accommodate that vision, and ensure that the seed does not die in her hand.

> **This women's ability to be a seed carrier goes beyond**

> **just being pregnant for nine months and giving birth to a child, it cuts across the man's visions, dreams, purpose, ambition, careers, vocations, and every other thing that can be birthed forth.**

The helper office of the woman comes into play in this her ability to be a seed carrier. Notice, the man has been with the seed, but it cannot bring forth fruits, no matter how hard he tried. Then he asked for help because he cannot bring forth without the women.

We are living in a world where people think that women have no specific assignment but just to help. Also, people believe that when you ask for help, it means that you are weak, and that is why most men tend to deny the fact that they need help, let alone asking for the help, just for them to be seen as superman.

I want you to sincerely answer me if you can do something by yourself, will you ask for help? There is this popular saying that states "Am I going to beg God to help me in what I know I can do?" So, it is very obvious that man needs help, no matter how he denies that fact. Even God himself knew that the man needs help and that is why He had to wire His omnipotence's into the women, for them to have all the ability to help.

It will be a disadvantage to the man if he refuses to ask for that help. And even if the man did not ask, for help, it does not still deny the fact that she is a help suitable.

> **God himself knew that the man need help and that is why He had to wire His omnipotence's into the women, for them to have all the ability to help.**

As a woman, you need to choose wisely when it comes to choosing the seed giver, because if you choose the wrong seed giver, he will certainly give you a wrong seed, and the bad effect of it is that the woman will still carry the seed and bring it forth. The woman is indeed a seed carrier, but what if the seed she received has been destroyed with all manner of vices, what if the seed has been destroyed with alcoholism, sexual immoralities, and the likes. That is why it is good to check if the seed you will bring forth is actually what you want to bring forth. This is why you will see innocent women bringing forth seeds that do not look like them. I am not talking about the physical appearance, but the character and other manifestations of the seed.

> **Choose wisely when it comes to choosing a seed giver because the wrong seed giver results in the wrong seed.**

God saw the man He has given the mandate to increase and multiply is still stunted, and showing no sign of growth. So, he had to intervene, by building up and making a creature that can carry and birth forth this mandate. He needed to be sure that His omnipotence has been built up in this creature so that there could be growth. When everything was now in place, He now paraded her before the man.

When God wanted to save humankind, He sought a woman that can carry and bring forth the seed of salvation. It was never a random selection; it was a very tedious one. God was looking for a woman that has not deviated from the principles been taught in the secret place. A carrier that has not been adulterated with vices, a carrier that will look like the seed. A carrier that has sustained the ability to dwell in the secret place. The search has been ongoing ever since Isaiah prophesied that the young virgin shall conceive and bear a Son. All the young virgins might have been asking themselves, "could it be me?" until finally a young virgin who was about preparing for her wedding received the salutation from Angel Gabriel; (Luke 1:28) *And having come in, the angel said to her, "Rejoice, highly favored one, the Lord is with you; blessed are you among women!"*

Finally, the long search was over. A carrier for the seed of salvation has been found. Now, what if this carrier for the seed of salvation has filled her life with all manner of immoralities and vices? What if she has given to testing before the wedding as is the norm of the day? The seed of salvation would have been delayed, even though there was nothing wrong with the seed.

We are currently living in a world where most young ladies have turned themselves into universal litmus paper for fertility. People no longer see the need to keep the matrimony bed sacred, most men want the lady to become pregnant for them to be sure that they can give birth before the wedding. We are living in a world where 98% of the married couples have tested and finished the honey in honeymoon and still claim to go for honeymoon after the wedding. We are living in a society where ladies are been used for sexual gratifications all in the name of relationships.

These days, most men have devised a way of getting the woman to dance to their tune by simply saying that they want to marry them. The devil has seen that seed of greatness that you are to carry and he has devised a strategy to corrupt the environment of that seed. Imagine putting a beautiful seed into a pool of acid, even though the seed needs liquid to grow, acid is never the best liquid. Imagine putting the beautiful seed in a room where immoralities have become the order of the day. Despite all the potentials for being good that is in the seed, the environment is also very essential for its growth.

Since it is good to choose the right seed giver, the carrier that provides the environment for the growth also needs to be preserved. You can imagine what could have been the fate of mankind if this carrier for the seed of salvation has deviated from the standard, if she has traded her purity for a few minutes' satisfaction. It was a serious search, imagine God seeing one generation pass, another came and also passed, yet He couldn't find any. Little wonder the angel said "blessed are you among women" that means that God has searched among the multitude of women, yet none passed the aptitude test.

The need for the carrier to preserve the environment of the seed is not something that happened and remained in the past, it is something that is still highly needed in today's world. God is still in the business of distributing great seeds, but His fear is the environment of the carrier, He is concerned about not putting the wonderful and fearfully made seed into acid or poison. He is concerned about the bird that may come to pick this wonderful seed, He is concerned about the rocky ground that may not be fertile enough to carry the seed till it brings forth its harvest, the thorns that can choke the life out of the beautiful seed.

Don't live your life casually, thinking that it will not affect the seed you carry. You cannot fill the environment of the seed with negativity and still expect to bring forth a seed that is filled with positivity.

Don't be deceived into thinking that God does not care about the environment of the seed, because He cares so much about it. Why do you think He will go to the extent of telling the seed carrier to stay away from a certain diet during the seed carrying? *(Judges 13:4-5); [4] Now, therefore, **please** be careful not to drink wine or similar drink, and not to eat anything unclean. [5] For behold, you shall conceive and bear a son. And no razor shall come upon his head, for the child shall be a Nazirite to God from the womb; and he shall begin to deliver Israel out of the hand of the Philistines.* Just look at how pathetic the instruction was, imagine God begging for something. Don't you think it is something that gives Him concern? If He can go the extra mile of pleading that the physical environment is maintained, how much more the spiritual environment!

Take, for instance, you are putting clean water into a dirty cup, no matter how neat the water maybe, just by mere putting it into the dirty cup changes the status of the water. This is just an analogy of what it means to put a fearfully and wonderfully made seed into a contaminated environment. Don't be deceived, if God is not concerned about the seed carrier, he wouldn't have pleaded.

EMBEDDED IN EVERY WOMAN, IS THE INTRINSIC ABILITY TO BE HIGHLY PERCEPTIVE.

Women by default are highly perceptive, they don't even struggle too much to have insight into any given situation. They understand perfectly what it means to think outside the box. Probably, it may be part of the omnipotence of God in them to bring out a solution to every problem in the course of their office as a helper. You can imagine how frustrating it can be when you have hope that someone can help you and the person couldn't offer such help. This is what God wanted to avoid by making the woman highly perceptive.

> **Women by default are highly perceptive, they don't even struggle too much to have insight into any given situation.**

Most men are ignorant of this perceptive nature of women and that is why some call them all manner of names, such as being too insecure or worrying about something that does not exist and even being overprotective. A wise man will grow this perceptive nature of the woman, and when it is been maximized, the home will be saved from avoidable errors and potential losses.

As a woman, you need to discover that this ability to be highly perceptive has been meticulously incorporated inside of you by God, and it will be an error when you could not offer much help when the need arises. You need to deal with the inferiority complex first because you need to be confident enough to convince someone to buy your idea. Most times, you know what to say to remedy the situation, but because you have self-doubt, and an inferiority complex, you just resort to keeping quiet and watching things go wrong.

> **As a woman, you need to discover that this ability to be highly perceptive has been meticulously incorporated inside of you by God, and it will be an error when you could not offer much help when the need arises.**

The man who is usually too goal-oriented, may not discover where there is a missing link. But the woman who usually pays close attention to every detail will easily discover such missing link even before it becomes obvious because of this intrinsic ability to be highly perceptive. I am not saying that women cannot be too goal-oriented, they can be too goal-oriented and still navigate any missing link because of this highly perceptive nature.

This highly perceptive nature of women can be seen even at a tender age, when compared with a male child of the same age, you will see that the verbal intelligence of the girl is usually higher than that of the boy. Women due to this their highly perceptive nature have more problem-solving abilities, appear smarter, more focused, and can effectively multi-task than men.

You can give a man and a woman the same task, when you compare both results you will see that the woman's own will look smarter. The reason is not farfetched the woman pays more attention to details than the men. This is not an avenue to feel superior or boast rather, it calls for total understanding and application of these abilities for the growth of society. Most men who tend to subdue these abilities in their wives are making a huge mistake because that was not the original intention of those abilities.

> **Women due to this their highly perceptive nature have more problem-solving abilities, appear smarter, more focused, and can effectively multi-task than men.**

EMBEDDED IN EVERY WOMAN, IS THE INTRINSIC ABILITY TO NURTURE.

The intrinsic ability of the woman to nurture does not just start when a woman gives birth to a child, it goes beyond that. It marvels me whenever I see little female children always displaying this nurturing ability effortlessly. They always want to protect their younger siblings, most times even to their detriments.

God has intrinsically configured the physiology of the woman in such a way that by default, it nurtures the seed right from the very moment of conception. The presence of the womb inside of a woman has already implicated her to nurture. This is why most times even when the woman is not present with the child, she can always perceive when things are not going well with the child or when the child is in danger.

Many women even prefer to be harmed than for anything to happen to the child. She does it unconsciously because this nurturing ability has been embedded in her. Despite how hardened, situations can make the heart of a woman be, it can never prevent her from displaying this nurturing ability.

This nurturing ability is what birth forth the mother in a woman. The ability to nurture is not restricted to only women who have given birth; mothers. It transcends beyond being a mother, which is why it is seen even in little female children.

This nurturing ability is what makes a woman extremely sacrificial, she can effortlessly give up things she needs for the sake of others. She can denial herself many things just to make sure that others are comfortable. It baffles me the extent a woman can go to protect and provide for those they nurture.

> **The presence of the womb inside of a woman has already implicated her to nurture.**

This is also the reason why they love without reservation. When a woman loves, she loves with everything in her, and it is quite unfortunate that most men have exploited this attribute of the woman negatively. This is why every woman needs to have an adequate understanding of this nature, to know when they are being negatively exploited and when they are not.

> **When a woman loves, she loves with everything in her, and it is quite unfortunate that most men have exploited this attribute of the woman negatively.**

You may be thinking that this nurturing ability of the woman is restricted to just nurturing children, but it is not so. They have the intrinsic ability to nurture the dream, potentials, and all manner of seeds. Things don't easily die in the hand of a woman. And the reason is that they have this intrinsic ability to nurture. They don't mind sacrificing all just to see that the seed is flourishing. Their joy comes from seeing the seed flourishing.

Any wise man can trust whichever seed he has into the hand of a woman because she knows how to nurture it till she sees the best. She has the intrinsic ability to protect such dreams from dying, all she needs is a collaborative and supportive effort.

> **This is time to locate and enter that place of unveiling and come out shouting eureka!**

The problem with most women today is that they don't even understand what is intrinsically configured in them. This is time to locate the key to that secret place where the knowledge of what is embedded in us are been locked up. This is time to enter that place of unveiling and come out shouting eureka! *(An exclamation indicating sudden discovery)*. This is time to maximize our God-given abilities as a woman because your generation is earnestly waiting for your full emergence and manifestation.

EMBEDDED IN EVERY WOMAN IS THE INTRINSIC ABILITY TO BE A WIFE

Being a woman gives you the leverage to become a wife, but that is not all to be a wife. Most women assume that being a woman automatically makes them a wife, but that is a costly assumption.

Remember Eve was first called a woman before being called a wife. Genesis 2:23 amp. *Then Adam said, This [creature] is now bone of my bones and flesh of my flesh; she shall be called Woman because she was taken out of a man.* The problem we are having today is that most women don't even understand their womanhood before looking for the title 'wife.' Most women are so obsessed with the idea of being a wife to the extent that it deprives them of their ability to be a woman. And the problem is that it only takes a whole woman to make a whole wife. When the woman fails to understand what it takes to be a woman, it also deprives her of the ability to be a wife and this has contributed to the reason why comparative terms have been added to the word 'wife.'

Most women are so obsessed with the idea of being a

> **wife to the extent that it deprives them of their ability to be a woman.**

The rate at which many women who pose to be a wife have gotten it wrong has made some adjectives like 'good' 'virtuous' 'capable' to be added before a wife. That was not so from the beginning. When the word 'wife' was first mentioned, it was just wife and no comparative terms, but because of the rate by which being a wife has been biased, there was now need for comparative terms which never solved the problem but gave rise to more problems.

> **The rate at which many women who pose to be a wife have gotten it wrong has made some adjectives like 'good' 'virtuous' 'capable' to be added before a wife.**

Genesis 2:24 amp. *Therefore a man shall leave his father and his mother and shall become united and cleave to his wife, and they shall become one flesh.* The place of the first mention of the word wife was just wife, but now any man that wants to marry will either tell you that he is looking for a good wife, some have even amplified it by saying that they are looking for a 'very good wife.'

We need to first become the woman that we are before looking for that which we can be. In an attempt to become that which we can be, most women have lost that which they are. A story was once told of a woman who burnt her boyfriend simply because he want to marry another woman. This woman in question might have not discovered who she is as a woman, had she discovered, she wouldn't have been desperate to marry that particular man. She wouldn't have seen it as though that is the end of the world for her. Probably she might have cleaved without being a wife.

> **We need to first become the woman that we are before looking for that which we can be.**

Most women today have become unmarriageable because they

have assumed the office of a wife before becoming one. And when the assumed husband or cohabiting husband now decides to marry a wife, the cohabiting wife will commit suicide or kill the cohabiting husband. Most women also, have subjected themselves to begging a man to marry them simply because they have freely occupied the office of a wife in the life of such a man and the man in question will not see any reason to marry, because all his need in a wife has been met.

> **In an attempt to become that which we can be, most women have lost that which they are.**

The office of the woman as a wife is only restricted to her husband. You can be a good woman and at the same time a bad wife. You can also be a perfect mother and at the same time be a bad wife. You can be a mother to a multitude of people, even to all nations, but you cannot be a wife to any other person apart from your husband. So as a woman, if you want to enjoy the office of a wife, you must deliberately decide to balance every area of your life so that no area suffers.

> **You can be a mother to a multitude of people, even to all nations, but you cannot be a wife to any other person apart from your husband.**

The reason why most marriages grow soar after the birth of the children is that most wives concentrate more on their children and ignore the husband with the assumption that he should understand. The truth is just that he is not understanding and you need to balance the gap before it leads to separation or two strange individuals living in the same house all in the name of marriage. This is the reason why you have to not just stop with the decision to be a wife but strategically plan on how to be a wife before becoming one.

Most women don't even understand what it means to be a wife

and that is why some will resort to being a mother in an attempt to be a wife. The ignorance of the wife has made most husbands jealous of their children, because the wife has transferred all her care and attention to the child, leaving little or no time for the husband.

◆ ◆ ◆

BEING A WIFE COMES WITH DECISION.

The fact that you are a woman, does not automatically make you a wife. Being a wife comes with the decision to be one. Life is designed in such a way that we make a decision about some things and as a woman, the decision to be a wife or not is part of some of the decisions you have to make in life.

It baffles me the way most women especially in the African continents are so eager to be married simply because most of their mates are been married to. Most of these women have not taken time to decide if they want to become a wife, at what time of their life they want to become a wife, what relevant knowledge is been needed before they become a wife, they are just so obsessed with the whole idea of being married to when their assumed mates are been married to.

This is the reason why you need to understand the times and seasons of your life and not judge your life with the times and seasons of others. The fact that a particular design may be trending does not mean that you are among those that the designer had in mind while designing it.

> **Life is designed in such a way that we make decisions about some things and as a woman, the decision to be a wife or not is part of some of the decisions you have to make in life.**

The earlier women understand that the prerequisite to be a wife is to first be a woman and when you are now a woman, you can then decide whether or whether not to become a wife the better for us. The problem is that society has made it look as though any person that is not a male will get married and become a wife, and this has configured the sense of desperation on the side of most females. Most people, especially in the African continent, don't even believe that one needs to decide to become a wife, they believe it is mandatory and this has made most women see becoming a wife as a do-or-die affair, get by all means issue. But it was never designed to be so.

Being a wife comes with the decision to cherish and give time to your husband despite your role as a mother. Being a wife comes with the decision to share your time with your husband, it comes with the decision to accept your mother-in-law and fathers-in-law like your own biological mother and father. It baffles me the way most women treat their mother-in-law and father-in-law. Some, especially those in the African continents call their mother-in-law names like "that witch" that old fool" "that dog" "that trouble maker" and all manner of names that are not called for. Some even prefer to marry someone whose parents are late simply because they are not ready to accept them as their biological parent.

Being a wife does not just end with deciding to be a wife. It also requires strategic planning of when and how to become a wife, it doesn't just end with mere wishes of deciding to be a wife, there is a doing aspect of becoming a wife.

◆ ◆ ◆

BEING A WIFE COMES WITH STRATEGIC PLANNING.

Planning is inevitable in our everyday life, even when you fail to plan, life also plans for you, but not to succeed but to fail. You need o strategically plan to be a wife because it will guide you in making the choice of whom to be married to, how to manage your home, and most importantly, how to be a wife.

This your plan must be SMART where:

S = Specific

You don't just want to marry any man. Before deciding on the specific area of concentration you need in a husband, you need to first discover your purpose and your direction in life. So, your plan must be specific; it should be well defined and devoid of ambiguity. Write out the things you want in the husband, is he someone that will be going in the same direction as you or someone who will take you away from your purpose? Is he someone that would want to swim when you want to fly? Is he someone that can bring out the good in you or is he someone that will kill it with compares and abuse?

> **Before deciding on the specific area of concentration you need in a husband, you need to first discover your purpose and your direction in life.**

The reason why most women struggle so much in choosing whom to marry it's that their plan if any, is generalized instead of being specific. The more generalized the plan is, the more difficult it is for you to easily arrive at a particular conclusion. Another reason is also that most have not discovered their purpose, and because they don't have any direction, they think that any road will lead them to their destination.

Some men are naturally confused, so when they see any signal that you are also confused, the wise ones will run for their dear life. When you have a direction, someone will even know where to start from. Not having direction is like standing at a bus stop waiting for a lift and when someone wants to offer help, you just quickly reply anywhere. Anywhere is simply nowhere. I believe you don't want to be referred to as someone who is going nowhere.

As a wife, you need to make a specific plan of how you want to balance your role as a mother, your role as a child of God (your spirituality), and your role as a wife. If you become so wonderful a mother and fail in the area of a wife, you have failed in your marriage. If you become a firebrand woman that commands heaven to fall, and it falls and then fails in the area of being a wife, you have failed God. So, there is a need to have a specific plan on how to balance your spirituality, motherhood, and the office of a wife to your husband.

> **As a wife, you need to make a specific plan of how you want to balance your role as a mother, your role as a child of God (your spirituality), and your role as a wife.**

Most families are in a mess today simply because the wife did not balance her role as a child, her role as a mother, and her role as a wife. Funny enough, most wives perfectly understand how to be spiritual, they perfectly understand how to be a mother, but rarely did they understand how to be a wife. And this is the reason why they think that anything can go in so long as they have a husband.

M = Measurable

You must have specific criteria that will measure your progress towards the accomplishment of your specific plan. Take for instance that you want to marry a university graduate, the measurable aspect of your plan could be from this range of graduation year, the courses studied, the grade they came out with and so many others.

When you eventually become a wife, what are some factors that you will put in place to monitor the progress of your specific plans? For instance, you planned to give birth to two children within five years of your marriage, after the fourth year you have given birth to one and you are also pregnant with the second child. At this point, you are making progress in the accomplishment of your plan. Or for instance, you have a specific plan of helping your husband become one of the top five employees in their firm after five years of your marriage, when you measure his current level after each year, you can determine the progress of your specific accomplishment and re-strategize when the criteria for measuring the progress is not giving you the desired result.

The essence of having a measurable specific plan is for you to monitor your progress and to re-strategize when the progress is not as expected. But when you don't have measurable criteria, it will be very difficult for you to determine whether you are making any progress or not.

> **The essence of having a measurable specific plan is for you to monitor your progress and to re-strategize when the progress is not as expected.**

A = Achievable/Attainable

The goals you hope to accomplish as a wife are they achievable or something impossible to achieve? Most women list all manner of qualities they want in a husband, most of which even them know that it is not achievable. Some will even list some qualities that can only be found in one person which is Jesus, and unless such plan is been re-examined, such woman will remain unmarried because Jesus is not looking for a wife.

Some women have decided to build a castle in the air which is not bad, but it is advisable to put a foundation under it. Going back to the choice of a husband, most people have narrowed it down to the point that the person will be one in one million people which invariably makes the possibility of the person being married to such a man very infinitesimal if at all possible.

The reason why God brought the woman to the man and not Adam is for her to choose among the numerous options available to her. But some women have so narrowed their plan that it must be Mr. A and when Mr. A is not forthcoming, they might end up chasing every other people away.

> **The goal and joy of every plan are to see it been achieved. It is a motivation to plan more.**

When the plan is not achievable it not only makes the plan void but also affects subsequent plans. It is good to aim high and widen your horizon when making plans, but also make it achievable.

The goal and joy of every plan are to see it been achieved. It is a motivation to plan more. So, when you plan and didn't achieve it because the plan is unachievable, it becomes a total waste of time and energy.

R = Realistic

The rate at which most young women makes unrealistic plan to be wife is quite alarming. A beautiful plan of how to be a good wife to your husband in heaven is unrealistic because wife and husband only exist here on earth.

The earlier you get rid of all those childish plans and face reality the better. As beautiful as building a castle is, it is very unrealistic when built in the air. Some women plan to be treated like a queen by their husbands, but they have not tried to be a queen. The earlier we come out of wishful thinking and face reality as it is. Some women are still under the illusion that their prince charming is coming to look for them without making realistic plans of acquiring relevant knowledge and skills that will make them visible to their prince charming.

Some women have made the plan of a husband who is not relevant to their life purpose. As good as such a plan may be, it is unrealistic if you truly want to fulfill the purpose. Some women have also planned to love every other person but their husband, as good as such a plan may be, it is unrealistic if you truly want to be a wife.

T = Timely

Any plan no matter how beautiful it may be without a clearly defined timeframe or timeline is unattainable. The reason why we attach a timeline to our plan is that we are living on a time-bound planet. It is also done to create urgency.

Time has always been in existence before man. To have a strategic plan, there is a need to attach a starting time and a target time. The starting time marks the beginning of the accomplishment, while the target time is set aside for the actualization of the plan.

When for instance you plan an event without attaching time to it people can come when the event has already been concluded. As a good planner, you need to attach a timeline to your plan, for example, you can state that from January 2022 to January 2023 that this is what I planned to achieve. You then create an urgency that will compel you to work round the clock to make sure that it is been achieved. In this case, January 2022 is the starting time while January 2023 is the target time.

> **The reason why you need to understand your time and season is that you need it in your planning.**

The reason why you need to understand your time and season it's because you need it in your planning. You cannot have the plan of what to do when you have not married to be the same when you are married. The reason why some women use the timing of others as their timing it's because they have not attached a timeline to their plan. You have indeed decided to be a wife, you still need to attach a timeline to it. For example, is it after high school, before high school, or during high school? When you attach a timeline to your plan, it helps you to prepare your spirit, soul, and body for that particular purpose.

As a wife, there is a need to attach a timeline to all your plans, you need to sit down with your husband and strategically write out all your plan attaching a timeline to them. For example, when to start giving birth to children, the number of children, how to create leisure time for yourselves, when to hang out with the whole family and when it will just be for you and your husband, and so many other examples. When you set out a particular time for a particular purpose, the accomplishment of such a purpose is already high. But when there is no timeline attached, you assume you can do it at any time, and anytime it's no time, which mostly renders such task unattainable.

> **The reason why some women use the timing of others as their timing it's because they have not attached a timeline to their plan.**

This planning to be a wife does not just end with short term plan that only exists till you are been married, it also involves a long-term goal/plan of what happens during the execution of the plan; when you are already a wife.

◆ ◆ ◆

BEING A WIFE IT'S A CALL TO LOVE

The primary duty of any wife to her husband is to love and care for him. As a wife you don't need to be reminded to love your husband, loving him is non-negotiable as long as you have decided to be his wife. Every other person you need to love is secondary when it comes to you occupying the office of a wife to your husband. This is a very hard nut to crack for most women.

> **You can be a daughter to your biological mother, mother-in-law, mentors, father, father-in-law, and many others, but you cannot be a wife to any other person aside from your husband.**

The reason why most wives struggle to love their husbands it's because they don't even understand why they are wives. You being a wife means that you are a wife exclusively because you have a husband. So, if you cherish the title of being called a wife, you should also cherish your husband, because you are a wife as a result of him marrying you. You can be a daughter to your biological mother, mother-in-law, mentors, father, father-in-law, and many others, but you cannot be a wife to any other person aside from your husband.

As a wife, you have to love your husband, mother-in-law,

your father-in-law, your brother and sister-in-law, your husband's relatives, and many others, but among all these people you have to love, your primary person to love is your husband. Other people are secondary, even your children as long as the office of a wife is the case study.

◆ ◆ ◆

BEING A WIFE IT'S A CALL TO BE SUBMISSIVE

Ephesians 5:22 amp. *Wives, be subject (be submissive and adapt yourselves) to your **husband** as [a service] to the Lord.* Ephesians 5:24 amp. *As the church is subject to Christ, so let wives be subject **in everything** to their husbands.*

The Bible has commanded the wife to be submissive to their husband. So, any woman that wants to occupy the office of a wife should be ready to submit to the husband. The command to be submissive it's non-negotiable in the life of every woman that has decided to be a wife.

Since it is non-negotiable to be submissive to your husband, you need to be very careful in choosing whom to submit to before marriage. You have the right to choose whom to submit to, but you don't have the right not to submit to your husband when you eventually marry him.

The problem most wives have with being submissive starts from their choice of a husband. They tend to choose a man who does not have a head, they tend to choose a husband that doesn't even know Christ let alone loving her as Christ loved the church, they tend to choose a man that cannot love to the extent of giving up themselves for the wife. Before the Bible command the wife to be subject to the husband, in Ephesians 5:22, it first commanded both the husband and wife to be subject to one out of reverence for Christ in Ephesians 5:21.

> **Since it is non-negotiable to be submissive to your husband, you need to be very careful in choosing**

> **whom to submit to before marriage.**

Someone once asked me if a man should submit to his wife and children, I referred him to Ephesians 5:21 where the Bible stated *"Be subject to one another out of reverence for Christ (the Messiah, the Anointed One)."* and Ephesians 5:25 amp. *Husbands, love your wives as Christ loved the church and gave Himself up for her.* If the husband has understood what it means to love to the extent of giving up oneself for the sake of the wife, what is being submissive that he cannot be? The problem is that most husbands don't even understand what it means to love as Christ did for the church.

> **The problem most wives have with being submissive starts from their choice of a husband.**

Most wife finds it difficult to submit to their husband because they don't love their husband. When you truly love someone, there is nothing you cannot do for such a person. The problem we have in our world today it's that virtually everyone claims to know what love is, but the truth is that out of all the people claiming to know what love is, only about 5 % of them truly understand what it means to love. And the truth of the matter is that you cannot give what you don't have.

Love it's the bedrock of every marriage and relationship, it's the active ingredient that fuels other facets of marriage. And whenever this love is lacking, it usually makes it difficult for other areas to stand the test of time. When it's lacking, wives struggle to submit to the husbands and the husband struggles to be subject to the wife.

> **Love it's the bedrock of every marriage and relationship, it's the active ingredient that fuels other facets of marriage.**

◆ ◆ ◆

BEING A WIFE IT'S A CALL TO COMFORT, ENCOURAGE, AND DO GOOD.

Proverb 31:12 amp. *She comforts, encourages, and does him only good as there is life within her.* So, as long as the wife lives, her duty toward her husband is to comfort, encourage, and do Good to the husband. The reverse has been the case in most homes as many wives instead of encouraging their husbands are now competing with them. Instead of making the home a comfortable place for the husband to rest, have made it a marketplace with their nagging.

Most wives instead of doing good to their husbands have deliberately decided to do him bad. Some will even say that they must deal with him, "does he think he can do this to me and go scot-free?" "I must repay him" "I must pepper him" all these and many more are the comment of most wives who are supposed to do good to their husbands.

Every human being is designed in such a way that they love comfort. The home is supposed to provide comfort for the dwellers, when this comfort is not been provided by the wife, the husband seeks it outside, and it will be so unfortunate for the wife if the husband finds this comfort outside. In this case, no matter how hard the wife tries, it will be very difficult for the husband to find that comfort in her again and most, it results in separation and divorce.

As a wife, you need to do everything possible to ensure that the home remains comfortable for the husband if you want a lasting marriage. The reason why you have to marry someone who is going towards the direction of your purpose, someone whom your purpose complements, it's for you to encourage him. You cannot encourage someone to do what you detest, which is the reason why you have to choose wisely and check compatibility tests before saying "I do."

Most women think that compatibility test is only done for the blood group and Rhesus factor, but the truth is that that is the easiest compatibility test to carry out as far as marriage is concerned. Blood group and Rhesus factor it's among the last compatibility test to check for. The first compatibility test to check after discovering that you both have the same Father should be on character, a test of honesty, sincerity, teach-ability, and many others should be positive because there are the things that will help you to do good to him as long as you live.

> **Most women think that compatibility test is only done for the blood group and Rhesus factor, but the truth is that that is the easiest compatibility test to carry out as far as marriage is concerned.**

Most women throw away all warning signals all in the name of love is blind. Who told you that love is blind? Are you the one that blindfolded the love or made it blind? If you so believe that love is blind, then marriage will cure the blindness for you and then, it will be too late. No husband suddenly starts being wicked, dishonest, or insincere after marriage, it has always been there but, because you were carried away by the euphoria of love, you didn't see the warning signals. Likewise, the most character displayed by the wife has always been there, but the husband threw away all the warning signals.

EMBEDDED IN EVERY WOMAN IS THE INTRINSIC ABILITY TO BE A MOTHER.

The fact that you are a woman does not automatically make you a mother. You don't choose to be a woman, but you choose to be a mother. But being a woman gives you the leverage of being a mother. You are first a woman before you become a mother, you cannot just be a mother without being a woman.

Any adult female human is called a woman, but any woman who gives birth to a child, raises a child, or has supplied her ovum for fertilization can be called a mother. But being a mother is all-encompassing and not restricted to the above definition.

> **The fact that you are a woman does not automatically make you a mother.**

There are different types of mothers, and different definitions of them based on how the role of mothers are defined culturally, religiously, and socially, which includes but is not restricted to:

1. **Biological Mothers:** any woman who may or may

not parent a child but has given birth to a child and has supplied her ovum for fertilization, can be called a biological mother. She has through sexual intercourse or egg donation genetically contributed to the creation of an infant, whether she decided to raise or parent the child or not.

2. **Adoptive Mothers:** any woman who by her raising a child, becomes a parent to the child through a legal process of adoption. This implies that you can be a mother even without giving birth or supplying an ovum for fertilization purposes.

3. **Stepmother:** here, the woman in question generally does not have the legal rights and responsibilities of a parent to the child/children, but by marrying the child/children's father, may form a family unit which now gives her the right to be called a mother.

4. **Surrogate Mothers:** a woman can be called a surrogate mother when she either gives birth to a child or provides her ovum for fertilization. There are two kinds of surrogate mothers which are:

   - Traditional Surrogate: where the father's sperm is artificially inseminated into the woman who then carries and delivers the baby for the partner that then takes up the responsibility of raising the child.
   - Gestational Surrogate: this is a medical technique generally referred to as 'in vitro fertilization; IVF'

Here, the mother is being referred to as the egg donor, she donates her egg which is then been fertilized with the sperm from the father; the sperm donor, the embryo is then placed into the uterus of a gestational surrogate who then carries the baby until the baby is been given birth to.

This gestational surrogate is called the birth mother while the biological mother is the woman who donated the egg that was fertilized.

◆ ◆ ◆

BEING A MOTHER COMES WITH DECISION.

We don't argue the fact that you are a woman, but you cannot just automatically become a mother simply because you are a woman. Most people think that being a woman automatically makes them a mother, but it's not true. Rather being a woman simply grants you access to become a mother if you choose.

In most African countries, they believe that all there is to be a woman is to become a mother. And that is why most parents especially the mothers become so obsessed with their daughter becoming a mother so that they can go for the postpartum care of the mother and her baby (popularly called "omugwo" "ojojo omo" "uwaan" in some parts of Nigeria's tribes). This is why the phrase 'when' you give birth instead of 'if' you give birth is popularly used in most African homes.

Being a mother comes with a decision, you must deliberately decide to be a mother before venturing into being a mother. Being a mother is not something that just happens accidentally, except in rare cases where there is a case of rape which eventually results in the victim becoming pregnant and then giving birth to the child.

Since being a mother comes with a decision. It then necessitates adequate preparation. There is this popular saying "that he who fails to plan, plan to fail" so, since you have decided to be a mother by the virtue of you being a woman, it does not still negate the fact that you need to plan for it.

> **Being a mother comes with a decision, you must deliberately decide to be a mother before venturing into being a mother.**

You cannot just say that because you are a woman, that you have known all there is to be a mother. After deciding to be a mother, the next thing is planning how to become an effective mother, the type of mother you want to become, and things you need to do to become such a mother.

❖ ❖ ❖

BEING A MOTHERS REQUIRES STRATEGIC PLANNING

With the decision to be a mother, comes the planning. The reason why most children do not get the best from their mothers it's because their mothers never took time to plan how to be a mother, they may probably be obsessed with the whole idea of being a mother and then forget the most important aspect which is the planning aspect.

Every stage of a woman's life needs proper planning, and any stage that you deliberately or ignorantly refused to plan for, the lapses will always show up. These lapses even become worst when other people are brought into the equation of your life, and most especially when it comes to being a mother. It is worst when it comes to being a mother because it gives birth to a generational problem that will take only the grace of God and strategic wisdom to correct.

> **Since you have decided to be a mother by the virtue of you being a woman, it does not still negate the fact that you need to plan for it.**

Our society is in a mess today simply because most women who consciously decided to be a mother, refused to plan on how to be a mother. So many young women today just think that all there is to be a mother is just to be a woman, and with this mindset, they don't see the need to plan for it. When this happens, the child will not be properly trained and the cycle keeps repeating from one generation to another. This results in bringing up children that cause a nuisance to society.

We are living in a world where most women see planning as something done by those who are jobless. And because they have this mindset of I am too busy, they see it as an absolute waste of time to sit down and plan for anything. They see planning as something that is not relevant and therefore, it can easily be eliminated from their day-to-day activities.

God never did any single thing without planning, it is evidenced in virtually every page of the bible. If God our creator never did anything without planning, then why can't we the creatures do the same? Since the fall of man, God has been planning on how to redeem mankind, it was never a day plan. When He was done with this plan, He made it known to mankind through the prophets, till He finally executed the plan strategically and mankind was saved.

> **Every stage of a woman's life needs proper planning, and any stage that you deliberately or ignorantly refused to plan for, the lapses will always show up.**

Most times your plans may not be strategic enough to achieve the desired goal, and in the case of deciding to be a mother, you can share the plan with your spouse, there is this wise saying "that two **good** head is better than one" emphases on the good. If there is a need to re-strategize the plan, the necessary adjustment can be done to bring forth a tremendous result.

The problem that some people that manage to plan mostly encounters is that the plan may not be clear enough to run with. You are mandated as a woman, not just to plan but to make the plan clear enough so that it can be properly understood and executed. When the plan is not strategic enough, the execution will be faulty, and this is why most people even after planning do not see a positive result.

> **If God our creator never did anything without planning, then why can't we the creatures do the same?**

It is important to note that the success of every strategic plan comes from God and this is why He is inevitable in every stage of the planning and execution. It is foolishness to ignore the chief planner in your plan. Most women do not involve Him in their plan, and when things go wrong which is always bound to happen whenever you do not involve Him, you start calling on Him to come and finish what He never stated.

This is time for us to deliberately decide not just to involve God in our plan, but to make Him the chief planner of our plans because we are a subset of His creative plan. He starts the formation of the child in your womb and continues the work until you put to birth, He now leaves the child under your care as a caretaker. But, it seems like most mothers are not happy or contented with the position of a caretaker for a child whom they carried for nine months or whom they are raising as the case may be. When the caretaker now suddenly decides to be the landlord/owner, there is usually a problem.

> **It is important to note that the success of every strategic plan comes from God and this is why He is inevitable in every stage of the planning and execution.**

Most mothers today have left their office as caretakers and are now struggling for ownership, and this is why most mothers have become adulterated owners of their children ignoring the original owner. And the result of this illegal ownership is usually disastrous.

Whenever any mother recognizes her place as the caretaker of her child, the duty of mothering the child becomes very easy and enjoyable. Do you know why? It is usually the landlord that takes the sole responsibility for the land. Your work as a caretaker is just to make sure that things are going smoothly and when there is any problem, you will report to the landlord who knows how best to handle the situation.

> **Whenever any mother recognizes her place as the caretaker of her child, the duty of mothering the child becomes very easy and enjoyable.**

For you to effectively plan to be a mother to any child, you need to go to the initiator of the child's existence and then discover from Him how and ways to continue His plan. This is because every human born of a woman already has days allotted to such individual, and has been deeply known and wonderfully crafted by God. Psalms 139:13. (*For You formed my inward parts; You covered me in my mother's womb*). And Psalms 139:16. (*Your eyes saw my substance, being yet unformed. And in your book they all were written, the days fashioned for me when as yet there were none of them*).

> **Having known that every single child has a blueprint, it then behooves on every woman who has decided to be a mother to find out the blueprint of her child. To work in line with God's original plan for the child.**

This Psalms 139:13 and 16 made it clear to us that no child is a biological accident, that each child already existed before the actual existence, and that God did not just plan in His mind, but rather, He documented our days and all that is expected of each day. Having known that every single child has a blueprint, it then behooves on every woman who has decided to be a mother to find out the blueprint of her child. To work in line with God's original plan for the child.

Whenever any mother does not get the blueprint of the child, the possibility of bringing up the child with a plan different from that which the original planner had in mind will be very high. You tend to bring up the child based on what you want, which may not be in line with what God wants the child to become. This is mostly the reason why most parents force their children into the wrong vocation simply because that is what is trending.

BEING A MOTHER IS A DEEP CALLING

You don't just decide to be a mother simply because you are a woman, not so. Being a mother it's a deep calling that should not be carelessly decided. It is not something that you just wake up one morning and decide to be or something that you decide to do simply because others are doing it. It is not something you just carelessly say that you feel like doing, it is a deep calling that goes beyond just feeling to be a mother.

> **Being a mother it's a deep calling that should not be carelessly decided.**

Women have been given a great privilege and opportunity by God to partner with Him in the area of giving life to another human being. Being a mother is something you prepare your spirit, soul, and body, emotions, psychology, mind, and many more to do. Being a mother is a vocation and needs to be treated as such. It is a vocation of love, it is a vocation that you have to give an account of. The reason why most women who have decided to be mothers do not make full proof of it is that they don't see it as a vocation, and as such, they take it as something they can just easily squeeze out of their busy schedule.

1. Being A Mother Is A Call To Love Unconditionally.

You are expected to love unconditionally when you decide to be a mother. As a mother, you don't just love because the receiver of the love did something spectacular, or because the child is always obedient, or because of any condition. As a mother, you love unconditionally.

It is this unconditional love of a mother that God has, that made Him love every one of His children irrespective of any bad record they might have had in the past. That is also what makes Him give rain to both the good and the bad.

It is this unconditional love of the mothers that makes them love all their children equally; both the good and the bad. The reason is that despite how bad the child may be in the eyes of others, just like God, they always see the good in them and that is what propels them to always love unconditionally.

> **As a mother, you don't just love because the receiver of the love did something spectacular, or because the child is always obedient, or because of any condition.**

Most children have withdrawn from being bad simply because of this unconditional love that they have received from their mothers. This is also the reason why most sinners get converted when they see the unmerited love of God despite their sinful life.

2. Being A Mother Is A Call To Be Compassionate.

Being compassionate is an attribute irreplaceable in the life of every woman who has decided to be a mother. Even when you tend to subdue this attribute, it will always showcase itself.

This attribute of being compassionate was directly embedded in them by God Himself, and it is evidenced in the life of Jesus whom the Bible repeatedly states in the whole four gospels that He had compassion on the crowd. In essence, He had compassion on His children, because being God, He sees the crowd like His children which brought out the compassion of a mother in Him and then made Him have compassion on them.

Any woman who has decided to be a mother and yet does not show compassion needs to be questioned because with the decision to be a mother comes the acceptance to be compassionate. Most women have ignored this compassionate attribute of mothers and this has led to so many errors in our society today, it has made many questions if such a woman is a mother.

> **Being compassionate is an attribute irreplaceable**

> **in the life of every woman who has decided to be a mother.**

This is a call for us to be compassionate, not just to our children but to society at large. Let us always try to see our children in other people's children and this will propel us to have compassion on them, and in the long run birth forth a society that will be conducive for the growth of all.

3. Being A Mother Is A Call To Nurture.

The intrinsic ability of women to nurture is made prominent in the lives of mothers. Women naturally can nurture, but when it comes to being a mother, the nurturing ability of the woman is being magnified and becomes more significant.

The quality of the nurturing offered by the mother is usually seen when the child is not with the mother. You can boldly say that you have nurtured properly when the recipient of the nurture can represent you in your absence. If the recipient of the nurture is only representing or doing well in your presence and the vice in your absences, then there are lapses somewhere that still need to be corrected by nurturing.

> **The quality of the nurturing offered by the mother is usually seen when the child is not with the mother.**

Life has been designed in such a way that whatsoever you sow, that you shall reap. And how you make your bed, so shall you lie on it. In nurturing, there is no room for mistakes because whichever mistake you make in the course of your nurturing, the child tends to grow with it.

Children by default tend to learn more from your nonverbal training than the verbal one. When you are telling them to do A with your mouth, but your action is communicating B to them, they may do the A in your presence but the B have subconsciously entered them.

Most times you may be wondering why your child is behaving in such a manner you did not verbally teach him or her, the reason is not farfetched, your nonverbal actions register more than the verbal ones.

> **Children by default tend to learn more from your nonverbal training than the verbal one.**

You may tell the child not to lie, but here you are lying to someone in his/her presence, tomorrow the child will lie to people.

The call of a mother to nurture is a very deep calling that demands everything in you; your time, love, understanding, wisdom, resources, and many other things. Since being a mother is a call to nurture, then you have to do it with all diligence, you have to be psychologically, emotionally, economically, socially, and spiritually ready to do so.

There is a reward for every good work, and whatever you invest in the cost of your nurturing, you always reap the reward. The nurturing ability demands that you will deny yourself so many things, it demands that you don't have to give up on the child, it demands that you bring up the child according to the stipulated pattern. It is in the nurturing of a child that the vocation of being a mother is made prominent and therefore, should never be joked with.

> **Since being a mother is a call to nurture, then you have to do it with all diligence, you have to be psychologically, emotionally, economically, socially, and spiritually ready to do so.**

If every child is well nurtured, then our society will take better shape. The problem is that most people who have decided to be mothers have failed in their ability to properly nurture their child. And the problem with these lapses is that these children who have not been properly nurtured tend to negatively influence the good ones giving rise to an increase in vices.

4. Being A Mother Is A Call To Selflessness.

We are living in a generation where me, my, mine, I, myself have become the words of the day. Everyone is seeking his or her good, we no longer have a common good anymore.

With the decision to be a mother comes the call to selflessness. You seek not just for your good but also for that of your child/children, family, and society. Because, if you seek just the good of yourself and that of your family ignoring that of the society you are living in, the selflessness is incomplete.

Being a mother is a call to selflessness because it is going to cost you your own life, you give up many things just for the sake of the child. You give up some habits just for the sake of the child. You deny yourself sleep just to make sure that the child is comfortable.

When our society embraces this selflessness of a mother, we will have a better society devoid of selfish people. The problem we have today is that most mothers don't embrace this selflessness of a mother, which is why some mothers despite being a mother watch someone's child die without offering a helping hand.

> **Being a mother is a call to selflessness because it is going to cost you your own life, you give up many things just for the sake of the child.**

This selflessness of a mother was being displayed by Mary the mother of Jesus, who when the angel delivered the message of how she will conceive and give birth to a son, offered herself for the sake of the child. She never considered how she will be mocked by her peers, the shame she is going to face, the stigma, and even her dismissal by her spouse, rather she offered herself without reservation. You can imagine what would have become of our salvation if she made a selfish decision if she considered her ego and status in society.

The attitude being displayed by some mothers has made people ask if they are mothers at all. The reason is that they have failed to embrace this selflessness of a mother. We are living in a world where most mothers have become even the most selfish people in the world. And that is not even the problem, the problem is that they transfer it to their children and the cycle keeps rotating.

AFTERWORD

REVIEW OF CHAPTER ONE

Chapter one lays great emphasis on The secret place.
What happened to the rib in the secret place?
So, the Lord God caused a deep sleep to fall upon the man, and he slept; then He took one of his ribs and closed up the flesh at that place (Genesis 2:21 NASB2020) You do recall that when God made them, he created them male and female; not male first and female later as most people misinterpret. God took a rib while Adam was fast asleep because he needed to spend time to create the woman in the secret place.

This chapter made me realize this part of the scripture I never considered intimately. God needed no distractions for the creation of Eve because she is a delicate creature and so are all women delicately made in the hands of the father. The Author managed to break down these secret place encounters into several subheadings you will read the same when you go through the book yourself. A secret place is a place of intimacy. It's a place made for two to share koinonia and fellowship. To have encounters and breed upon life and goals.
This is why the secret Place is:
1. A place of formation: It is in the secret place that the woman discovers the reason for which she is made. God said it is not good for a man to be alone. This is a core part of the manufacturer's guide. If I may say, manual. Most young women drift away from this path and are mishandled and carelessly maltreated because they haven't

◆ ◆ ◆

REVIEW OF CHAPTER THREE

I consider it a great privilege to be doing a review of WOMBMAN by Ogechi Obayi; and particularly review of chapter 3 titled: The Concept 'Time' This chapter was beautifully written to the woman aspiring to achieve the best of God for her. I believe this chapter also works well with men who have goals to achieve before them.

The story of the five foolish or "other virgins" as described by the author does justice to this chapter. They corrected their mistakes, got extra oil, alas, the doors were shut. The value of timeliness cannot be overemphasized.

Things to look out for in this chapter
• Principle of timing: Time counts whether you choose to count it or not.
• Value of understanding times and seasons: The sons of Issachar were leaders because they knew times and seasons.
• Plans and timeliness: Make hay while the sun shines because if you do not... You know what can come after it.
• Preparation and Opportunities: Manifestation comes when preparation meets opportunity.
• Maximizing Opportunities: Discipline and giving it all it takes. You must be ready for the discomfort growth brings.
Questions to ask yourself for you to maximize this book:
• What are my goals?
• What should I be doing now?
• What sacrifices should I make for my next level?
If you do these, then I tell you have made good use of what the author has in mind. I believe this is a book to read and you should avail yourself of the opportunity of getting the book.

Dr. Jegede Ayodapo Oluwadare
(Lecturer, Fellow of West African Postgraduate College of Pharmacists, Educator at the foundation for a drug-free world and currently the resident Pastor at Kings Word International Church Ile-Ife).

REVIEW OF CHAPTER FOUR

He made me a woman and the anchor Scripture is Genesis 2:22
From this chapter which is made up of seven pages, I was able to extract eight (8) major points that the author pharmacist Ogechi did a good job at making. Briefly:

1. The fact that the building up of a woman happens in a secret place. I will like to take us back to the scripture; in Genesis 1:27 God made male and female, however in this place Genesis 2:22 God now built up a woman. You will notice that a female has always been in existence from the time of creation; God made them male and female. After that process, God took a rib from the man and then made a woman, and that point was what Ogechi was trying to x-ray; the fact that God took the rib and nobody knows what He did with the rib, the only thing we saw was the end product of that building up, and it happened in the secret place. So, as women, we cannot overemphasize the place of the secret place, the place of intimacy, the place of communion, the place of koinonia with God, because that is where the making and building up happens. A female remains a female until she goes to the secret place and becomes a woman.

2. The importance of the woman having a thorough understanding of the woman she is. This understanding is very important because it will make her see her worth and it will make her quit struggling for a place of importance with the man in the family or society. A woman who knows her worth will see that she is not in any way inferior to a man, but she is different, she is a man with huge addition which is the womb and hence the title of the book 'Wombman.' And that addition of the womb in this man (so, a woman was first and foremost a man, however, she is a man that has a womb), makes it possible for the woman to give birth and be able to nurture another life. So that the woman now shares this character with God; the ability to bring forth life, and also to be able to nurture this life. And a woman can do this in a very unique way because it is God-given and that is why this woman is the good of the man, the family, and society. So that when a woman understands this privilege; this ability to make a difference in the family, in the life of another man, and the society at large, she will see that she is not in any way disadvantaged being a woman.

3. That while God formed a man, He 'built' a woman. It may seem to be the same but reading commentary on this verse of the Bible made me understand that the forming and the building up of man and woman respectively make a huge difference to the end product. Implying that God gave huge attention to the process of making a woman, it didn't just happen overnight and that is why the transformation of being just a female to a woman takes time. When God wants to transform you and when you are yielded to become a woman in its full sense, it takes time. It's not something that just occurs, it takes time. It's a transformation process.

4. God was not in a hurry at all while making women, because it was a transformation process. And this chapter made us understand that in this

process, God had to even put Adam to sleep so that He will have the full attention and concentration in making this special type of man.

5. God performed the first wedding between 'the man and the woman'. According to Pharmacist Obayi in this fourth chapter, God after making a woman presented her to the man and not Adam. And this is seen by some as the first wedding ceremony which was done by God; God was the officiating Priest of this wedding ceremony between the man and the woman. And the reason why God presented the woman to the man and not the woman to Adam was to show that the marriage institution was something that will go beyond Adam and Eve; something that has come to stay, and what will continue to be even till the end of the world. So, the woman was presented to the man and that started the marriage institution.

6. God put Adam to sleep so He could build up a woman without being disturbed. She also pointed out that as women, it is our duty to go back to God to understand who we are, it's not for a man to tell us who we are, because he was not there during the making. She is saying in this chapter four, that we do not do ourselves any favor when we wait for a man to make us know our worth. Yes, the men can help when used by God however, the person who knows how best to do it the best is God because He was the one that made us in the secret place, He made us become women and by going back to Him to help us understand what happened to build us up, we will understand who we are, our worth, and be able to maximize that worth as women.

7. The Woman is the updated version and last edition of God's creation.

8. The last point I was also able to extract in the fourth chapter is the point that Ogechi was trying to make when she talked about a woman making Jesus cry, from that I understood that: Women are deeply emotionally connected to God. And that can achieve a lot for the woman herself, the man, and the society at large. Because women as the last born of creation, as she put it, we have this deep connection with God which we are meant to maximize.

The author concluded that chapter by emphasizing the need for women to be able to understand their worth because that is the only way they will be able to live out their full potential on earth, it will also help them to stop struggling to be what they are not and start maximizing that which they are. And with that, she concluded that chapter and as a person, I have learned so much and I hope that as you pick up this book to read, God will also reveal things about you personally, things that He has built into you that you are yet to see so that you will be able to maximize them and live out your full potential on earth.

Thank you for the opportunity to review this book, it is a privilege.

Dr. Chinazom Precious Agbo
(Lecturer in the Department of Pharmaceutics and an award-winning Researcher, she has co-authored a good number of publications in peer-reviewed journals, she is a lover and chaser of God).

$$\blacklozenge \quad \blacklozenge \quad \blacklozenge$$

REVIEW OF CHAPTER FIVE

IS BEING A WOMAN A DISADVANTAGE?
I thank our sister Ogechi, for doing a great job on this book. This book came on time. The subheading of chapter five is a kind of a question. This question arises as a result of the way we women are moving about as though we just woke up from our slumber after a very long time of being suppressed, and realizing that we are been suppressed by men, then coming out we are now coming out in such a way that we are now trying to take what has been deprived of us for a long time. Being a woman in the actual sense is not in any way a disadvantage, the Bible told us that is God that made everything, and after creating every other thing, He created male and female, and no one of them is more important than the other, we are to complement each other, but not to compete. So, in women coming out to take their place in society, they are now doing it in such a way as if they are rubbing shoulders with the men, trying to compete, but it is not so.
These are the points I was able to extract from chapter five of this book:

Our culture in the African part of the world has contributed a lot to seeing being a woman as a disadvantage. Before now, women are deprived of so many opportunities, such as access to good education, the pursuit of their careers which they could have competently handled with other roles ascribed to them by nature. Today women are coming up to take their places in society. This doesn't call for competition with men. Bible said God created them male and female with different features and responsibilities. Though none is superior to the other. They are to complement each other and not to compete. The role of a woman should be played with discretion.

In this case, there is a call by the author for every woman to discover what it takes to be a woman and appreciate that responsibility. It's easier for women to discover who they are and become that, than trying to become who they are not. Unfortunately, this issue of women trying to be like men and not appreciating themselves has its root in their mothers, who were not well informed and in turn, can't give what they don't have. The Author, therefore, calls on all women to be who they are meant to be, this will make them satisfied as well as their maker. God has equally given women all it will take to fulfill this responsibility. Women are also called not to repeat the mistakes of the past.

By **Recommendations**

This book is a must-read for every woman of any age. Not just for every woman alone, it is also for all men, because every man has a woman as a daughter, as a wife, as a sister, and as a mother. So that we all shall come out as the author our sister Ogechi said to correct this mistake that we've made in the past.

Once again, I say thank you so much for considering me worthy to be a part of your wonderful work.

Mrs. Chikaodili Igbokwe
(A member of supervising world; a global multinational company, a marriage, and relationship coach, and a counselor).

◆ ◆ ◆

REVIEW OF CHAPTER EIGHT

EMBEDDED IN EVERY WOMAN IS THE INTRINSIC ABILITY TO INFLUENCE
1. The first miracle performed by Jesus was as a result of the influential power of a woman.

With a heart full of gratitude to the Almighty God, I appreciate our beloved sister in Christ Jesus, Ogechi Obayi for this deep and revelational, heartwarming, and spirit-powered exposition. Sincerely, intrinsic in every woman is embedded varieties of ABILITIES.

The author, in this chapter, raised and exposed beautifully the INFLUENTIAL ABILITY of every woman. "Any woman, no matter the age or size has the intrinsic ability to influence any man; despite his age." The above quote is heavy and controversial but was accurately dissected and exposed by the author.

The author integrated sufficient ideas and interesting events of life to reveal the influential ability of every woman. My eyes were open to discover how great the woman is and how careful we need to be before her. Reading this book with the heart to learn will trigger a more intuitive understanding of the beauty of man and woman as creatures of excellence.

However, it is significant to know that the influential ability of every woman is coefficient on the heart attitude of the woman.

A godly woman will influence men into godliness.

A worldly woman will influence men into worldliness.

A satanic woman will influence men into Satanism.

A canal woman will influence men into carnality.

In Summary, the author opens our hearts to understand how much we can trust women and how much we can be careful of them. **For whatever she carries, she sells.** Meaning that if men are not careful, a woman can sell a wheelchair to a man who is not lame. What a great book in this age of sex dilemma. I recommend this book to every man and every woman for a better understanding of human sexuality and its peculiar cum cooperative abilities. It will help the woman to discover and maximal her influential potential. It will also aid every man to accept the great endowment of influence in every woman and also learn how to maximize her influential potential without acting foolishly.

Mr. Johnpaul Marcilinus Ezema
(A teacher of teachers, certified Mathematician, vast in the experience of life, a Christian in attitude and words).

◆ ◆ ◆

REVIEW OF CHAPTER NINE

It's a privilege to be part of the reviewers of this great book and I must commend Pharm. Obayi for putting up this great piece at this kairos moment. Chapter 9 talks about the SEED CARRYING POTENTIAL OF WOMEN.

Obayi lets us know that in every woman lies the potential to be a seed carrier... an exclusive prerogative of Women! We are not just seed carriers, we are seed nurturers! We may have no say in the gender representation of the seed, but we determine its destiny. Women are powerful... we determine the future of the next generation. God has placed in us a precious mandate of securing the next generation via the godly act of conception, pregnancy, and child-rearing all through adulthood. It is an intentional process that must be reverently carried out. The bible says in Gen. 3:15 that the seed of the woman shall bruise the head of the serpent (paraphrased). Little wonder the popular rhetoric..."The future is female"

We must rise to our God-given mandate and play our part in sending the devil out of our Nation by raising and nurturing godly seeds. We as women must be intentional about this process of incubation because it is a great assignment and privilege to nurture divine seeds. If we leave it to chance, then we have left it to decadence. The "Wombman" which is the woman carries the potential of incubating the next generation. We are not just carrying seeds, we are carrying nations.

It is important to note; the quality of the seed is directly proportional to the quality of the seed giver. In the author's words: "Choose wisely when it comes to choosing a seed giver because the wrong seed giver results in the wrong seed"

Recommendation: I recommend this book for every woman, young couple, and girl teenager

Mrs. Chioma Peculiar-Onyekere
(She is committed to raising excellent youths that will stand out for God, she is passionate about youth excelling in their chosen careers while upholding Godly virtues).

◆ ◆ ◆

REVIEW OF CHAPTER TWELVE

I have the privilege to review chapter twelve of this very wonderful book with the sub-topic: Embedded in every Woman is the intrinsic ability to be a wife. Pharmacist Ogechi has made us understand that being a woman is a prerequisite to becoming a wife, but not a guarantee to be a wife. Ogechi reminded us also, that in Genesis 2:23 that Eve was first called a woman before she became the wife of Adam.

Interestingly, these first nuggets captured my fancy and I'm sure it will do the same to you, it states: most women are so obsessed with the nomenclature of wife that it deprives them of their first existence as women. Wow! And she says that that is why most of them have failed in the very high office of wifedom. And because of that, I'm sure today you hear somebody tell you I want a virtuous wife, I want a good wife. That adjective has become necessary to qualify the word wife. But Ogechi is telling us that being a wife is complete on its own and doesn't need any kind of cajoling or embellishments, because it is complete on its own if we do understand what it is.

Ogechi said that you can be a mother of the multitude, or even an entire nation without actually being a wife. Ogechi insists that being a wife is a deliberate decision that comes with strategic planning; on how to function as a wife, as a mother, and as a child of God. Ogechi also told us in chapter twelve, that this plan has to be SMART because it has to be Simply, it has to be Measurable, it has to be Achievable, it has to be Realistic, and there must be Time attached to it. Because if you understand your time, there will be no need for anxiety.

Ogechi further went on to say that being a wife, is a call to love, it is a call to submissiveness, it is a call to comfort and encouragement. Ogechi went further to look at the scenario where this day's people get married, and they are busy acting out what is happening at house A or house B, how wife A or wife B is behaving, and not going back to look at the drawing board of the family, which they would have done together as husband and wife to know what their timing is. Because if that has happened, definitely there wouldn't be any need for anxieties at one point or the other.

With every sense of responsibility, I would **Recommend** this book to all medical adults, medical adults as we say as pharmacists are those who are from twelve years and above.

Kudos to you, Pharmacist Ogechi Obayi, I know that this is a little peck into the future of a character that will come to great fulfillment in this country. Ladies and gentlemen, thank you very much, I consider it a great privilege to be asked to review this chapter twelve.

Pharm. (Mrs.) Ijeoma Okey-Ewurum
(An outstanding public speaker, delivered papers locally and internationally, a Behavioral change coach, and Author; the first book was published in 1994).

◆ ◆ ◆

Thank you for reading WOMBMAN: The good of a Man, Family, and Society.

You can reach out to the Author for review:

Phone number: +2348160307922

Email Address: obayicharityogechi@gmail.com

ACKNOWLEDGEMENT

I sincerely wish to acknowledge the Holy Spirit my chief source of inspiration. My parents, siblings, Uncles, and aunties for all their care and support. With a grateful heart, I humbly appreciate Mr. Theophilus Ndubisi and the entire Noble Ladies World because of the program that propelled me to start and finish this book. I also appreciate all my Mentors who have directly or indirectly shaped my life for good.
I sincerely appreciate all the reviewers of this life-changing book, you are the best.

ABOUT THE AUTHOR

Ogechi Charity Obayi

Is a young Pharmacist, a passionate Researcher and Writer, a Peer Moral Sex Educator, an e-creator and publisher, a Data Analyst, and a Graphic Designer. She is passionate about the youth maximizing their potentials, healthy relationships, and most especially young women discovering and maximizing their intrinsic abilities as women.